GIANT CELL ARTERITIS

DIET COOKBOOK
FOR BEGINNERS

Nourishing Recipes with Expert Guidance to Combat
Inflammation and Boost Your Health

Kingsley Klopp

Table of Contents

Fish and Seafood Recipes

Poultry Recipes

To show our appreciation for your purchase, we're delighted to offer you these special bonuses as a heartfelt thank you.

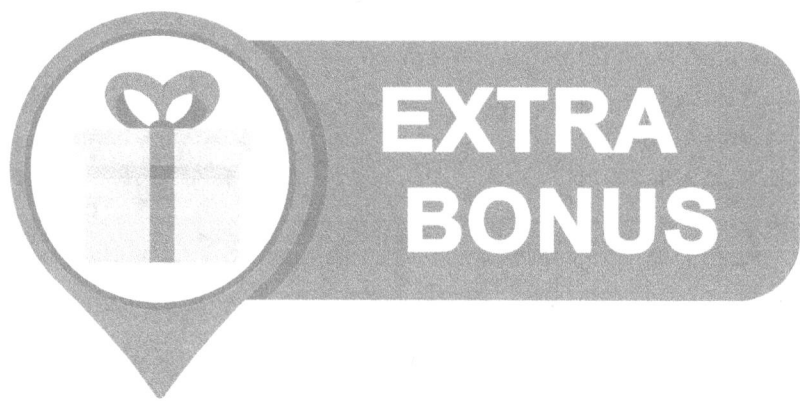

1. A Food Tracker Journal
2. Downloadable E-BOOK featuring full-color images of finished recipes

Important Note

This cookbook is a labor of love, crafted to help you navigate the challenges of Giant Cell Arteritis with a variety of nutritious and enjoyable recipes. However, as we set forth on this culinary adventure together, we must share an important note with you. Every individual is unique, and so are their dietary needs. While this cookbook is designed to offer meals that support the management of Giant Cell Arteritis, it's crucial to remember that what works for one person may not be ideal for another. We encourage you to listen to your body and make adjustments to the recipes as needed. You might find that certain ingredients work better for you or that you need to avoid others due to personal preferences or sensitivities. Flexibility is key. Don't hesitate to substitute ingredients or modify cooking methods to suit your needs. Your well-being is the priority, and your diet should reflect that.

Moreover, managing Giant Cell Arteritis often requires a tailored approach, and this extends beyond the kitchen. It's always a good idea to consult with your healthcare provider or a registered dietitian, especially if you have any questions or concerns about your diet. They can provide personalized advice that aligns with your overall treatment plan and health goals.

We also want to note that the nutritional information provided for each recipe is approximate. Variations in ingredients, brands, and preparation methods can influence the final nutritional content of a dish. While we strive for accuracy, these numbers should serve as general guidelines rather than exact figures.

Furthermore, If our cookbook has brought joy to your kitchen and table, we'd be thrilled to hear about your experiences in an Amazon review. On the flip side, if you stumble upon any hiccups while exploring our recipes, don't hesitate to get in touch at **kloppkingsley@gmail.com.**

In closing, we hope this cookbook serves as a helpful tool in your health journey, offering inspiration and guidance as you explore the wonderful world of anti-inflammatory foods. Remember to enjoy the process, savor the flavors, and above all, listen to your body.

Introduction.

Welcome to the **Giant Cell Arteritis Diet Cookbook for Beginners,** your essential guide to managing Giant Cell Arteritis (GCA) through delicious and nutritious meals. Whether you've just been diagnosed with GCA or are seeking new ways to improve your diet and overall health, you've taken a significant step toward better well-being by opening this book. Imagine this: a life where you wake up each day feeling more energized, with reduced inflammation, and better control over your symptoms. A life where food is not just a necessity but a powerful tool that helps you combat the challenges of Giant Cell Arteritis. This cookbook is designed to make that vision a reality. Through carefully crafted recipes and a comprehensive understanding of how diet impacts GCA, you'll discover how to transform your eating habits and improve your quality of life.

But first, let's take a moment to understand what Giant Cell Arteritis is and why diet plays such a crucial role in managing it. Giant Cell Arteritis is an inflammatory disease that primarily affects the arteries in your head. It can cause severe headaches, jaw pain, and even vision problems. The inflammation associated with GCA is not just painful but can lead to serious complications if not properly managed. This is where your diet comes into play.

Inflammation is a key player in the progression of GCA, and what you eat can significantly influence your body's inflammatory response. By choosing foods that have anti-inflammatory properties, you can help reduce the overall inflammation in your body, alleviate symptoms, and support your treatment plan. Conversely, avoiding foods that exacerbate inflammation is equally important to keep your condition under control.

Now, you might be thinking, "Does this mean I have to give up all my favorite foods and stick to a bland, restrictive diet?" Absolutely not! The "Giant Cell Arteritis Diet Cookbook for Beginners" is here to show you that eating for health can be both enjoyable and delicious. This book is packed with a variety of recipes that are not only beneficial for managing GCA but also bursting with flavors that will make every meal a delight. From hearty breakfasts that kickstart your day with energy to comforting soups and stews that warm your soul, this cookbook covers all bases. You'll find recipes for every meal of the day, including snacks and desserts that satisfy your cravings without compromising your health. Each recipe is crafted with carefully selected ingredients that fight inflammation and promote overall wellness.

What sets this cookbook apart is its focus on simplicity and accessibility. We understand that living with GCA can be challenging enough without the added stress of complicated meal preparations. That's why every recipe in this book is designed to be easy to follow, with straightforward instructions and readily available ingredients. You don't need to be a culinary expert to create these dishes – all you need is a desire to improve your health and enjoy good food. Moreover, this cookbook is not just about recipes. It's about empowering you with knowledge. You'll find valuable information on the role of different nutrients in managing GCA, tips on meal planning, and advice on how to make sustainable dietary changes. We want you to feel confident in your food choices and inspired to take control of your health through diet.

So, whether you're a seasoned cook or a kitchen novice, this cookbook is your companion on the journey to better health. Dive into these pages with an open mind and a ready palate. Discover the joy of eating well while managing Giant Cell Arteritis. Let's embark on this culinary adventure together, one delicious bite at a time. Welcome to the start of a healthier, happier you!

Chapter 1: Introduction to Giant Cell Arteritis

What is Giant Cell Arteritis?

Giant Cell Arteritis (GCA) is a complex and often misunderstood condition, shrouded in both mystery and significance. It is a form of vasculitis, which is essentially an inflammation of the blood vessels. However, GCA specifically targets the large and medium-sized arteries, particularly those around the temples, making it a critical condition that requires immediate attention and management.

The Silent Storm Within

Imagine the blood vessels as the highways of your body, responsible for transporting essential nutrients and oxygen to various organs. GCA is like a silent storm that brews within these highways, causing them to swell and narrow. This swelling restricts the blood flow, leading to a cascade of complications. The impact of this condition can be profound, affecting not only the physical well-being but also the emotional and psychological health of those diagnosed.

Historical Background

The first detailed descriptions of what we now know as Giant Cell Arteritis date back to the early 20th century. In 1932, the renowned pathologist Horton and his colleagues provided the initial clinical and pathological characterization of this disease, hence the alternative name "Horton's disease." Their pioneering work laid the foundation for understanding this enigmatic condition.

However, GCA has likely been a part of human history long before it was formally identified. Ancient medical texts hint at symptoms that could be attributed to GCA, showcasing how this condition has silently persisted through the ages, impacting countless lives.

The Emotional Toll

Receiving a diagnosis of Giant Cell Arteritis can be an emotional rollercoaster. The uncertainty and fear of what lies ahead can be overwhelming. This condition often strikes individuals over the age of 50, a time when many are looking forward to enjoying the fruits of their labor and spending quality time with family and friends. Instead, they are faced with a new challenge, one that disrupts their plans and forces them to navigate an unfamiliar medical landscape.

The Pathophysiology: A Closer Look

At the core of GCA is an immune system gone awry. In a healthy body, the immune system acts as a guardian, protecting against infections and other threats. In GCA, however, this guardian becomes misguided and turns against the body's own tissues. The exact cause of this autoimmune response is still a topic of ongoing research, but it is believed to involve a combination of genetic predisposition and environmental triggers.

When the immune system attacks the arterial walls, it leads to the formation of giant cells—large, multinucleated cells that are a hallmark of this condition. These cells, along with other inflammatory cells, create granulomas that cause the arterial walls to thicken. As the inflammation progresses, the arteries become narrow and even occluded, severely restricting blood flow.

The Impact on Daily Life

Living with Giant Cell Arteritis is a daily battle. The chronic pain and fatigue can make even simple tasks seem insurmountable. The need for frequent medical appointments and the side effects of long-term medication add to the burden. Yet, amid these challenges, many individuals demonstrate incredible resilience and strength. They adapt, find new ways to engage with their passions, and often become advocates for raising awareness about GCA.

Treatment and Hope

The journey of managing GCA is not one to be taken alone. It requires a comprehensive approach involving healthcare professionals, support groups, and loved ones. The primary treatment involves corticosteroids, which help to reduce inflammation and prevent complications. In recent years, advancements in medical research have introduced additional therapies, offering hope for better management of the disease.

Symptoms and Diagnosis

Common Symptoms

1. Headache: The most common symptom of GCA is a persistent, severe headache, often located at the temples. This headache can be described as throbbing or stabbing and may be accompanied by tenderness in the scalp.
2. Jaw Claudication: Pain in the jaw when chewing or talking is another hallmark symptom. This occurs due to reduced blood flow to the muscles of the jaw, making it difficult to perform even basic tasks like eating.
3. Vision Problems: GCA can lead to serious vision issues, including blurred vision, double vision, or even sudden, permanent vision loss in one or both eyes. This is due to inflammation of the arteries that supply blood to the eyes.
4. Scalp Tenderness: The scalp may become extremely tender to the touch, making it painful to comb hair or even rest your head on a pillow.
5. Fatigue and General Malaise: Patients often experience profound fatigue, a general feeling of being unwell, and sometimes unexplained weight loss.
6. Muscle Pain and Stiffness: Many individuals with GCA also have polymyalgia rheumatica, which causes pain and stiffness in the shoulders, neck, and hips, especially in the morning.
7. Fever: Low-grade fevers can occur, adding to the overall feeling of illness.
8. Night Sweats: Some patients experience night sweats, which can be drenching and disruptive to sleep.

Less Common Symptoms

1. Hearing Loss: While less common, some patients report hearing issues, including loss of hearing or ringing in the ears (tinnitus).
2. Tongue and Throat Pain: Pain in the tongue or throat can occur, particularly when swallowing.
3. Peripheral Neuropathy: Numbness, tingling, or pain in the limbs due to nerve involvement is another possible but less common symptom.

The Importance of Timely Diagnosis

Diagnosing GCA promptly is critical to prevent serious complications such as blindness or stroke. The diagnosis involves a combination of clinical evaluation, laboratory tests, and imaging studies.

Diagnostic Process

1. Clinical Evaluation: The initial step in diagnosing GCA involves a thorough clinical evaluation. A healthcare provider will take a detailed medical history and perform a physical examination, focusing on symptoms like headache, jaw claudication, and vision problems.
2. Blood Tests: Blood tests are an essential part of the diagnostic process. Elevated levels of certain markers of inflammation, such as the erythrocyte sedimentation rate (ESR) and C-reactive protein (CRP), can indicate the presence of GCA. These tests, while not specific to GCA, help to support the diagnosis when clinical suspicion is high.
3. Imaging Studies: Advanced imaging techniques are increasingly used to aid in the diagnosis of GCA. Ultrasound of the temporal arteries can show characteristic changes such as thickening of the artery walls. Magnetic resonance imaging (MRI) and positron emission tomography (PET) scans can also be useful in visualizing inflammation in larger arteries.
4. Temporal Artery Biopsy: The gold standard for diagnosing GCA is a temporal artery biopsy. This procedure involves taking a small sample of the temporal artery to examine under a microscope. The presence of giant cells and inflammation in the arterial walls confirms the diagnosis. Although highly specific, a negative biopsy does not completely rule out GCA, especially if clinical suspicion remains high.
5. Ophthalmologic Examination: Given the risk of vision loss, an ophthalmologic examination is crucial. An eye doctor may conduct various tests to assess the health of the eyes and the blood vessels supplying them.
6. Comprehensive Assessment: A comprehensive assessment may also involve consulting with rheumatologists, neurologists, and other specialists to rule out other conditions that might mimic GCA symptoms.

Emotional and Psychological Impact

Receiving a diagnosis of GCA can be overwhelming. The fear of potential complications, coupled with the chronic nature of the disease, can lead to significant emotional and psychological stress. It is important for patients to seek support from healthcare providers, family, friends, and support groups. Counseling and mental health services can also be beneficial in managing the emotional aspects of the condition.

Moving Forward with a Diagnosis

While a diagnosis of GCA is life-altering, it is also a gateway to managing the condition effectively. With appropriate treatment, many people with GCA lead full, active lives. Early diagnosis and intervention are key to preventing serious complications and improving the overall quality of life for those affected.

Treatment Options for Giant Cell Arteritis

Giant Cell Arteritis (GCA) is a serious condition that requires immediate and effective treatment to prevent severe complications, such as blindness or stroke. While the diagnosis of GCA can be daunting, the treatment landscape has evolved significantly, offering hope and improved quality of life for those affected. Here, are the various treatment options available for managing GCA.

Immediate Goals of Treatment

The primary goals in treating GCA are to reduce inflammation, alleviate symptoms, prevent complications, and improve overall well-being. This involves a combination of medications, lifestyle changes, and supportive care.

Corticosteroids: The Mainstay of Treatment

1. Prednisone: The cornerstone of GCA treatment is corticosteroids, with prednisone being the most commonly prescribed. Prednisone works by rapidly reducing inflammation, providing relief from symptoms such as headache, jaw pain, and vision disturbances. Treatment usually begins with a high dose, which is gradually tapered over time to the lowest effective dose.

2. Dosing and Tapering: The initial dose of prednisone is typically between 40-60 mg per day. This high dose is maintained until symptoms are controlled and inflammatory markers (ESR and CRP) are normalized. The tapering process can take several months to years, depending on individual response and disease activity.

3. Side Effects: Long-term use of corticosteroids comes with potential side effects, including weight gain, osteoporosis, high blood pressure, diabetes, and increased risk of infections. Patients are closely monitored for these side effects, and measures such as calcium and vitamin D supplements, bone density scans, and blood pressure monitoring are implemented to mitigate risks.

Adjunctive Therapies

1. Methotrexate: For some patients, especially those who require high doses of prednisone or have frequent relapses, an additional immunosuppressive medication like methotrexate may be prescribed. Methotrexate helps to reduce the steroid dose needed and maintain remission.

2. Tocilizumab: Tocilizumab, an interleukin-6 (IL-6) receptor antagonist, has emerged as a significant advancement in GCA treatment. Approved by the FDA for GCA, tocilizumab can be used in combination with corticosteroids or as a monotherapy. Clinical trials have shown that it can effectively reduce disease activity and steroid dependence.

Non-Pharmacological Approaches

1. Lifestyle Modifications: Patients are encouraged to adopt a healthy lifestyle to support their overall treatment plan. This includes a balanced diet rich in anti-inflammatory foods, regular exercise to maintain cardiovascular health and muscle strength, and smoking cessation.
2. Bone Health: Due to the risk of osteoporosis from long-term steroid use, patients are advised to engage in weight-bearing exercises and take calcium and vitamin D supplements. Bone density should be monitored regularly, and medications such as bisphosphonates may be prescribed to protect bone health.
3. Cardiovascular Health: Managing cardiovascular risk factors is crucial for GCA patients. This includes controlling blood pressure, cholesterol levels, and diabetes. Regular cardiovascular check-ups and a heart-healthy diet are essential components of care.

Monitoring and Follow-Up

1. Regular Assessments: Continuous monitoring is vital in managing GCA. Regular follow-up appointments with healthcare providers are necessary to track disease activity, adjust medications, and monitor for side effects.
2. Blood Tests: Frequent blood tests to measure ESR and CRP levels help assess the effectiveness of treatment and detect any signs of relapse. These tests provide valuable information about the inflammatory status of the patient.
3. Vision Monitoring: Given the risk of vision loss, regular ophthalmologic evaluations are critical. Any new or worsening visual symptoms require immediate medical attention.

Managing Relapses

Despite treatment, some patients may experience relapses where symptoms return or worsen. Early identification and intervention are crucial to manage these episodes effectively. Treatment strategies for relapses may involve increasing the corticosteroid dose temporarily or adjusting adjunctive therapies.

Psychological Support

The emotional and psychological impact of GCA should not be underestimated. The chronic nature of the disease, along with the side effects of long-term medication, can take a toll on mental health. Psychological support through counseling, support groups, and stress management techniques can significantly enhance the quality of life for GCA patients.

Research and Future Directions

Ongoing research continues to explore new treatment avenues for GCA. Clinical trials are investigating additional biologic agents and novel therapies that target specific pathways involved in the disease process. Advances in understanding the genetic and immunological aspects of GCA hold promise for more personalized and effective treatments in the future.

The Role of Diet in GCA Management

Giant Cell Arteritis (GCA) is more than just a medical condition; it's a life-altering journey that demands a holistic approach to management. While medications are essential, the role of diet in managing GCA cannot be overstated. For those living with GCA, diet becomes a powerful tool, a beacon of hope, and a source of strength in their daily lives.

Nourishing the Body, Nurturing the Soul

Food is more than sustenance; it is a way to connect with our bodies, nourish our souls, and empower ourselves to face the challenges of GCA. Every meal is an opportunity to fight inflammation, boost energy, and improve overall well-being. Understanding the impact of diet on GCA can transform how we approach this condition, making it possible to reclaim control and lead a vibrant life.

The Anti-Inflammatory Diet: A Foundation for Healing

At the heart of dietary management for GCA is the anti-inflammatory diet. Chronic inflammation is the root cause of GCA, and combating this inflammation through food can significantly aid in managing symptoms and improving quality of life.

1. Fruits and Vegetables: Bursting with vitamins, minerals, and antioxidants, fruits and vegetables are the cornerstone of an anti-inflammatory diet. Leafy greens like spinach and kale, colorful vegetables like bell peppers and carrots, and fruits such as berries and citrus fruits help to neutralize harmful free radicals and reduce inflammation.

2. Healthy Fats: Incorporating healthy fats into the diet is crucial. Omega-3 fatty acids, found in fatty fish like salmon and mackerel, flaxseeds, and walnuts, have potent anti-inflammatory properties. Olive oil, avocado, and nuts are excellent sources of monounsaturated fats, which also contribute to reducing inflammation.

3. Whole Grains: Whole grains like quinoa, brown rice, and oats provide essential fiber and nutrients that support digestive health and stabilize blood sugar levels. Unlike refined grains, whole grains have anti-inflammatory benefits and help maintain energy levels throughout the day.

4. Lean Proteins: Protein is vital for maintaining muscle mass and overall strength, especially for those on long-term corticosteroid treatment, which can lead to muscle wasting. Opt for lean sources of protein such as chicken, turkey, beans, and legumes to support muscle health without contributing to inflammation.

5. Herbs and Spices: Nature's pharmacy is rich with herbs and spices that possess anti-inflammatory properties. Turmeric, ginger, garlic, and cinnamon not only add flavor to meals but also help to reduce inflammation and support the immune system.

Foods to Avoid: Reducing the Inflammatory Load

Just as important as the foods to include are the foods to avoid. Certain foods can exacerbate inflammation and undermine the efforts to manage GCA effectively.

1. Processed Foods: Highly processed foods, laden with trans fats, refined sugars, and artificial additives, are pro-inflammatory and should be minimized. These foods include sugary snacks, fast food, and packaged meals.
2. Refined Carbohydrates: White bread, pastries, and sugary cereals can spike blood sugar levels and promote inflammation. Opting for whole grain alternatives can make a significant difference.
3. Red and Processed Meats: These meats are high in saturated fats and can increase inflammation. Limiting consumption of red meat and avoiding processed meats like sausages and bacon can help manage inflammation.
4. Sugary Beverages: Sodas, energy drinks, and sweetened teas are high in sugar and can contribute to inflammation. Staying hydrated with water, herbal teas, and natural fruit juices is a healthier choice.

The Emotional Impact of Dietary Choices

Living with GCA involves navigating a landscape of uncertainty and challenge, but making mindful dietary choices can provide a sense of empowerment and control. Each meal prepared with care is a step towards healing and resilience. Sharing nutritious meals with loved ones, exploring new recipes, and finding joy in the kitchen can be therapeutic and uplifting.

Practical Tips for Dietary Management

1. Meal Planning: Planning meals ahead of time ensures that healthy, anti-inflammatory options are always available. Batch cooking and preparing meals in advance can reduce the stress of daily cooking and ensure consistent adherence to a healthy diet.
2. Grocery Shopping: Creating a shopping list filled with whole, unprocessed foods can help make healthier choices easier. Sticking to the perimeter of the grocery store, where fresh produce, meats, and dairy are typically located, can also minimize the temptation of processed foods.
3. Mindful Eating: Paying attention to how and what we eat can enhance the benefits of a healthy diet. Eating slowly, savoring each bite, and listening to the body's hunger and fullness cues can improve digestion and overall satisfaction with meals.

Chapter 2: Nutritional Guidelines for GCA

Essential Nutrients for GCA Patients

Omega-3 Fatty Acids

Why They Matter: Omega-3 fatty acids are renowned for their potent anti-inflammatory properties. They play a crucial role in reducing inflammation, which is at the heart of GCA.

Sources: Fatty fish such as salmon, mackerel, and sardines are excellent sources of omega-3s. Plant-based sources include flaxseeds, chia seeds, and walnuts.

Incorporating Omega-3s: Aim to include fatty fish in your diet at least twice a week. Add flaxseeds or chia seeds to smoothies, cereals, or salads to boost your intake.

Vitamin D

Why It Matters: Vitamin D is essential for bone health and immune function. Long-term corticosteroid use, common in GCA treatment, can lead to bone density loss, making vitamin D crucial for maintaining strong bones.

Sources: Sunlight is a primary source of vitamin D, but it can also be found in fortified foods like milk, orange juice, and cereals. Fatty fish and egg yolks are natural sources.

Incorporating Vitamin D: Spend some time in the sun daily, and include vitamin D-rich foods in your diet. Consider supplements if you have a deficiency, but always consult with a healthcare provider first.

Calcium

Why It Matters: Like vitamin D, calcium is vital for bone health. Corticosteroids can lead to osteoporosis, so ensuring adequate calcium intake is critical for preventing bone fractures.

Sources: Dairy products such as milk, cheese, and yogurt are rich in calcium. Non-dairy sources include leafy greens like kale and broccoli, almonds, and fortified plant-based milks.

Incorporating Calcium: Aim for a balanced diet that includes a variety of calcium-rich foods. If necessary, supplements can help meet your daily calcium needs.

Antioxidants

Why They Matter: Antioxidants help to combat oxidative stress and inflammation, supporting overall immune health and potentially reducing GCA symptoms.

Sources: Fruits and vegetables are the best sources of antioxidants. Berries, oranges, spinach, and bell peppers are particularly high in these beneficial compounds.

Incorporating Antioxidants: Strive to fill half your plate with fruits and vegetables at each meal. Snack on berries or carrots, and add spinach or kale to smoothies.

Fiber

Why It Matters: A high-fiber diet supports digestive health and can help control weight, which is important since corticosteroid use can lead to weight gain.

Sources: Whole grains like oats, quinoa, and brown rice, as well as fruits, vegetables, beans, and legumes, are excellent sources of fiber.

Incorporating Fiber: Choose whole grains over refined grains, and include a variety of fiber-rich foods in your daily meals. Start your day with a high-fiber breakfast like oatmeal with fruit.

Protein

Why It Matters: Protein is essential for maintaining muscle mass, especially important for GCA patients on long-term corticosteroids, which can cause muscle wasting.

Sources: Lean meats like chicken and turkey, fish, beans, legumes, nuts, and seeds are good sources of protein.

Incorporating Protein: Include a source of protein at every meal. Opt for lean meats and plant-based proteins to keep your diet balanced and nutritious.

Magnesium

Why It Matters: Magnesium plays a role in bone health, muscle function, and reducing inflammation. It's also important for energy production and overall well-being.

Sources: Leafy green vegetables, nuts, seeds, whole grains, and legumes are rich in magnesium.

Incorporating Magnesium: Add a variety of magnesium-rich foods to your diet. Consider snacking on nuts and seeds, and include leafy greens in your meals.

B Vitamins

Why They Matter: B vitamins, particularly B6 and B12, support energy production, brain health, and red blood cell formation. They can also help combat the fatigue often experienced by GCA patients.

Sources: Whole grains, meat, eggs, dairy products, and legumes are good sources of B vitamins. Fortified cereals can also help meet your needs.

Incorporating B Vitamins: Eat a balanced diet that includes a variety of foods rich in B vitamins. Consider fortified foods if you follow a plant-based diet.

Zinc

Why It Matters: Zinc supports the immune system and helps with wound healing and DNA synthesis. It can also aid in reducing inflammation.

Sources: Meat, shellfish, dairy products, nuts, seeds, and legumes are rich in zinc.

Incorporating Zinc: Include zinc-rich foods in your diet regularly. Shellfish like oysters and crab, as well as meat and dairy, can help meet your zinc needs.

Foods to Include in Your Diet

Fruits and Vegetables: The Nutrient Powerhouses

Why They Matter: Fruits and vegetables are loaded with vitamins, minerals, antioxidants, and fiber, all of which are crucial for reducing inflammation and supporting overall health.

Top Choices:

1. Berries: Blueberries, strawberries, and raspberries are rich in antioxidants like anthocyanins, which help fight inflammation.
2. Leafy Greens: Spinach, kale, and Swiss chard are high in vitamins A, C, and K, as well as magnesium and iron, which support immune function and reduce inflammation.
3. Cruciferous Vegetables: Broccoli, Brussels sprouts, and cauliflower contain sulforaphane, an anti-inflammatory compound.
4. Colorful Vegetables: Bell peppers, carrots, and beets are packed with antioxidants like beta-carotene and vitamin C.
5. Citrus Fruits: Oranges, grapefruits, and lemons are excellent sources of vitamin C, which boosts the immune system.

Incorporating Them: Aim to fill half your plate with fruits and vegetables at each meal. Add berries to your morning cereal, enjoy a leafy green salad for lunch, and include a variety of colorful vegetables in your dinner.

Whole Grains: Sustained Energy and Fiber

Why They Matter: Whole grains provide essential fiber, vitamins, and minerals, helping to stabilize blood sugar levels and support digestive health.

Top Choices:

1. Quinoa: A complete protein that contains all nine essential amino acids.
2. Brown Rice: High in fiber and magnesium, which helps reduce inflammation.
3. Oats: Rich in beta-glucans, which have immune-boosting properties.
4. Barley: Contains soluble fiber that supports heart health.
5. Whole Wheat: Provides B vitamins and fiber for sustained energy.

Incorporating Them: Replace refined grains with whole grains in your meals. Enjoy oatmeal for breakfast, use brown rice or quinoa as a base for salads, and choose whole wheat bread and pasta.

Healthy Fats: Essential for Reducing Inflammation

Why They Matter: Healthy fats, particularly omega-3 fatty acids, have strong anti-inflammatory properties and are crucial for brain and heart health.

Top Choices:

1. Fatty Fish: Salmon, mackerel, sardines, and trout are excellent sources of omega-3 fatty acids.
2. Nuts and Seeds: Walnuts, flaxseeds, chia seeds, and almonds provide healthy fats and fiber.
3. Avocado: Rich in monounsaturated fats, which help reduce inflammation.
4. Olive Oil: Contains oleocanthal, an anti-inflammatory compound.

Incorporating Them: Include fatty fish in your diet at least twice a week. Add nuts and seeds to salads and yogurt, use avocado as a spread or in smoothies, and cook with olive oil.

Lean Proteins: Building and Repairing Tissues

Why They Matter: Protein is essential for muscle maintenance and repair, especially important for those on long-term corticosteroids, which can lead to muscle wasting.

Top Choices:

1. Chicken and Turkey: Lean sources of protein with minimal saturated fat.
2. Fish and Seafood: Besides being high in omega-3s, they are also excellent sources of lean protein.
3. Beans and Legumes: Black beans, lentils, and chickpeas provide plant-based protein and fiber.
4. Tofu and Tempeh: Great plant-based protein options, especially for vegetarians and vegans.

Incorporating Them: Include a source of lean protein at each meal. Grilled chicken or fish for dinner, beans or lentils in soups and salads, and tofu or tempeh in stir-fries.

Dairy or Dairy Alternatives: Bone Health Support

Why They Matter: Dairy products provide calcium and vitamin D, essential for bone health, particularly important for those on corticosteroids which can lead to osteoporosis.

Top Choices:

1. Low-Fat or Fat-Free Dairy: Milk, yogurt, and cheese offer calcium and vitamin D with less saturated fat.
2. Fortified Plant-Based Milks: Almond, soy, or oat milk fortified with calcium and vitamin D.

Incorporating Them: Include dairy or fortified alternatives in your daily diet. Enjoy yogurt with fruit for breakfast, use milk in smoothies, and add cheese to salads and casseroles.

Herbs and Spices: Nature's Anti-Inflammatories

Why They Matter: Many herbs and spices have anti-inflammatory properties and can enhance the flavor of your meals without added salt or sugar.

Top Choices:

1. Turmeric: Contains curcumin, a powerful anti-inflammatory compound.
2. Ginger: Known for its anti-inflammatory and digestive benefits.
3. Garlic: Has anti-inflammatory and immune-boosting properties.
4. Cinnamon: Helps regulate blood sugar and has anti-inflammatory effects.
5. Oregano and Thyme: Rich in antioxidants and anti-inflammatory compounds.

Incorporating Them: Add turmeric and ginger to smoothies, soups, and stews. Use garlic in cooking, sprinkle cinnamon on oatmeal or yogurt, and season dishes with oregano and thyme.

Hydration: Essential for Overall Health

Why It Matters: Staying hydrated supports all bodily functions, helps manage side effects of medications, and maintains overall health.

Top Choices:

1. Water: The best source of hydration.
2. Herbal Teas: Provide hydration without caffeine.
3. Natural Fruit Juices: Offer vitamins and hydration, but should be consumed in moderation due to natural sugars.
4. Water-Rich Foods: Cucumbers, watermelon, and celery add hydration and nutrients.

Incorporating Hydration: Drink at least 8 glasses of water a day, more if you are active or in hot weather. Include herbal teas and water-rich foods in your diet.

Foods to Avoid

Processed and Packaged Foods

Why They Matter: Processed foods are often high in unhealthy fats, sugars, and artificial additives, all of which can contribute to inflammation.

Examples:

1. Fast Food: Burgers, fries, and fried chicken are typically high in trans fats and unhealthy oils.
2. Packaged Snacks: Chips, cookies, and crackers often contain trans fats, high levels of sodium, and preservatives.
3. Pre-packaged Meals: Microwave dinners and instant noodles usually contain high levels of sodium, preservatives, and artificial flavors.

Reasons to Avoid: These foods can increase inflammatory markers in the body and contribute to weight gain, making it harder to manage GCA symptoms.

Sugary Foods and Beverages

Why They Matter: High sugar intake can lead to increased inflammation, weight gain, and can negatively impact blood sugar levels.

Examples:

1. Sugary Snacks: Candy, cakes, pastries, and donuts.
2. Sugary Beverages: Sodas, energy drinks, sweetened teas, and flavored coffees.
3. High-Sugar Cereals: Breakfast cereals with added sugars.

Reasons to Avoid: Excessive sugar consumption can spike blood sugar levels, leading to insulin resistance and increased inflammation. It also contributes to weight gain, which can complicate GCA management.

Refined Carbohydrates

Why They Matter: Refined carbs are stripped of their fiber and nutrients, leading to rapid spikes in blood sugar levels and increased inflammation.

Examples:

1. White Bread: Bread made from refined white flour.
2. White Rice: Polished rice that has had its fiber-rich husk removed.
3. Pasta: Especially when made from refined white flour.
4. Pastries and Baked Goods: Often made with white flour and added sugars.

Reasons to Avoid: Refined carbohydrates can lead to blood sugar spikes and crashes, contributing to inflammation and making it harder to manage GCA symptoms.

Saturated and Trans Fats

Why They Matter: These unhealthy fats can increase cholesterol levels and promote inflammation in the body.

Examples:

1. Red and Processed Meats: Beef, lamb, sausages, and hot dogs.
2. Full-Fat Dairy Products: Whole milk, butter, cheese, and cream.
3. Fried Foods: French fries, fried chicken, and other deep-fried foods.
4. Margarine and Shortening: Often contain trans fats.

Reasons to Avoid: High intake of saturated and trans fats can increase LDL (bad) cholesterol, contribute to heart disease, and promote inflammation, which is detrimental for GCA patients.

Excessive Salt (Sodium)

Why It Matters: High sodium intake can lead to water retention and high blood pressure, both of which can complicate GCA management.

Examples:

1. Processed Meats: Bacon, ham, deli meats, and sausages.
2. Canned Foods: Soups, vegetables, and beans often have added salt.
3. Salty Snacks: Chips, pretzels, and salted nuts.
4. Restaurant and Takeout Foods: Often prepared with high amounts of salt.

Reasons to Avoid: Excessive salt intake can lead to high blood pressure and fluid retention, which can exacerbate GCA symptoms and overall health.

Artificial Additives and Preservatives

Why They Matter: Additives and preservatives can trigger inflammatory responses and allergic reactions in some individuals.

Examples:

1. Artificial Sweeteners: Aspartame, sucralose, and saccharin found in diet sodas and sugar-free products.
2. Colorings and Flavorings: Artificial colors and flavors in candies, snacks, and beverages.
3. Preservatives: BHA, BHT, and sulfites used in packaged foods.

Reasons to Avoid: These substances can contribute to inflammation and may trigger adverse reactions, making it harder to manage GCA symptoms.

Alcohol

Why It Matters: Alcohol can interfere with the effectiveness of medications and increase inflammation in the body.

Examples:

1. Beer: High in calories and can contribute to weight gain.
2. Wine and Spirits: Can increase inflammation and interact negatively with medications.

Reasons to Avoid: Alcohol consumption can lead to increased inflammation, disrupt sleep patterns, and interfere with medication efficacy, complicating the management of GCA.

Gluten (for some people)
Why It Matters: Some individuals with GCA may also have gluten sensitivity or celiac disease, which can exacerbate inflammation.
Examples:
1. Wheat: Bread, pasta, cereals, and baked goods made with wheat flour.
2. Barley and Rye: Found in some cereals, bread, and beer.
Reasons to Avoid: For those with gluten sensitivity or celiac disease, consuming gluten can lead to increased inflammation and digestive issues, complicating the management of GCA.

Hence, avoiding certain foods is a crucial aspect of managing Giant Cell Arteritis. Processed and sugary foods, refined carbohydrates, unhealthy fats, excessive salt, artificial additives, alcohol, and gluten (for some) can all contribute to increased inflammation and complicate the management of GCA. By being mindful of these foods and making healthier choices, individuals with GCA can better manage their symptoms, reduce inflammation, and improve their overall quality of life. The journey to managing GCA is deeply personal and unique, but every mindful choice brings you one step closer to living a healthier, more empowered life.

Importance of Hydration in Managing Giant Cell Arteritis

The Role of Hydration in the Body

Water is the primary component of the human body, making up about 60% of body weight. It is involved in almost every physiological process, including:

- Regulating body temperature
- Maintaining electrolyte balance
- Facilitating digestion and nutrient absorption
- **Lubricating joints**
- Removing waste and toxins through urine and sweat
- Supporting cellular functions

For individuals with GCA, maintaining optimal hydration is crucial due to the added demands placed on the body by inflammation and medication.

Reducing Inflammation

Why It Matters: Inflammation is a hallmark of GCA, and proper hydration can help modulate the body's inflammatory response.

How It Helps: Staying hydrated ensures that cells function efficiently, and helps maintain the integrity of the mucous membranes, which act as barriers to pathogens and irritants. Hydration can also help flush out toxins and inflammatory by-products that accumulate in the body.

Supporting Medication Efficacy and Reducing Side Effects

Why It Matters: Medications, particularly corticosteroids, are a cornerstone of GCA treatment but can have significant side effects.

How It Helps: Hydration aids in the metabolism and excretion of medications, reducing the risk of side effects such as kidney stones and urinary tract infections. It also helps in preventing dry mouth and gastrointestinal discomfort, common side effects of some medications.

Enhancing Circulation

Why It Matters: GCA affects the blood vessels, leading to inflammation and narrowing that can impede blood flow.

How It Helps: Proper hydration ensures that blood is adequately viscous, promoting smoother circulation. This helps in delivering oxygen and nutrients to tissues more efficiently and can potentially alleviate some of the symptoms associated with GCA, such as headaches and muscle pain.

Maintaining Joint Health

Why It Matters: Joint pain and stiffness are common in GCA patients, particularly those who also have polymyalgia rheumatica.

How It Helps: Hydration keeps the cartilage in joints soft and flexible, reducing friction and wear. It also ensures that the synovial fluid, which lubricates the joints, is at optimal levels, helping to reduce pain and improve mobility.

Supporting Digestive Health

Why It Matters: Digestive issues can be a concern for GCA patients, especially those on long-term medication.

How It Helps: Water aids in the digestion and absorption of nutrients, as well as in the prevention of constipation by keeping stools soft and easier to pass. This is particularly important for individuals taking medications that can cause gastrointestinal side effects.

Preventing Fatigue and Enhancing Energy Levels

Why It Matters: Fatigue is a common symptom of GCA, exacerbated by inflammation and medication side effects.

How It Helps: Dehydration can lead to fatigue and decreased cognitive function. By maintaining proper hydration, energy levels are supported, and the body's ability to cope with stress and inflammation is improved.

Promoting Healthy Skin

Why It Matters: Skin health can be affected by both GCA and the medications used to treat it.

How It Helps: Adequate hydration helps maintain skin elasticity and moisture, reducing dryness and irritation that can be exacerbated by corticosteroids. This contributes to overall comfort and well-being.

Practical Tips for Staying Hydrated

1. Drink Water Regularly: Aim to drink at least 8 glasses (about 2 liters) of water daily. Increase intake if you are active, live in a hot climate, or are experiencing increased symptoms.
2. Eat Water-Rich Foods: Incorporate foods with high water content into your diet, such as cucumbers, watermelon, oranges, and strawberries.
3. Monitor Hydration Levels: Pay attention to signs of dehydration, such as dark urine, dry mouth, and dizziness. Aim for light yellow urine as a good indicator of adequate hydration.
4. Carry a Water Bottle: Keep a water bottle with you throughout the day to remind yourself to drink regularly.
5. Set Reminders: Use phone apps or alarms to remind yourself to drink water, especially if you tend to forget.
6. Herbal Teas: Incorporate herbal teas into your routine. They can be a flavorful way to increase fluid intake without caffeine.
7. Limit Dehydrating Beverages: Reduce consumption of caffeinated and alcoholic beverages, as they can contribute to dehydration.

Breakfast Recipes

1. Baked Avocado Eggs
Servings: 2
Cooking Time: 20 minutes
Ingredients
- 1 large avocado, halved and pitted
- 2 large eggs
- Salt and pepper to taste
- 1 tablespoon chopped fresh chives (optional)
- 1 tablespoon chopped fresh parsley (optional)
- 1 tablespoon grated Parmesan cheese (optional)

Instructions
1. Preheat your oven to 425°F (220°C).
2. Scoop out a bit of the avocado flesh to make room for the egg. Reserve the scooped avocado for another use.
3. Place the avocado halves in a small baking dish or on a baking sheet.
4. Crack an egg into each avocado half. Season with salt and pepper.
5. Bake in the preheated oven for about 15 minutes, or until the egg whites are set but the yolks are still runny.
6. Remove from the oven and sprinkle with fresh chives, parsley, and grated Parmesan cheese, if using.
7. Serve immediately.

Nutrition Info (per serving)
- Calories: 250
- Protein: 9g
- Carbohydrates: 6g
- Fat: 21g
- Fiber: 7g
- Sugars: 1g
- Sodium: 100mg

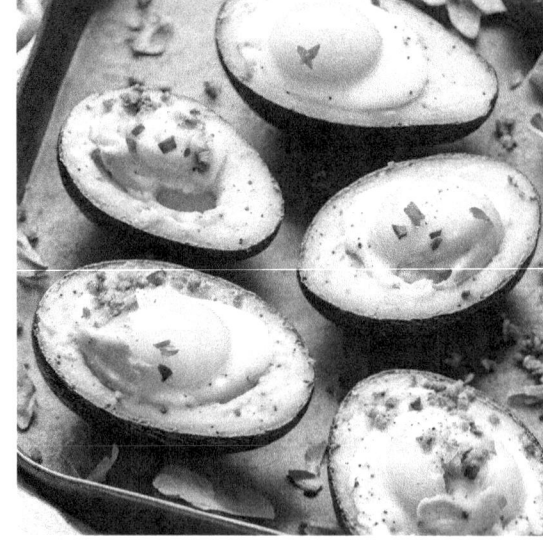

2. Avocado and Egg Breakfast Pizza

Servings: 4
Cooking Time: 20 minutes
Ingredients

- 4 whole grain pita breads or flatbreads
- 1 large ripe avocado, mashed
- 4 large eggs
- 1 cup cherry tomatoes, halved
- 1/4 cup crumbled feta cheese
- 1 tablespoon olive oil
- Salt and pepper to taste
- Fresh basil leaves for garnish

Instructions

1. Preheat your oven to 400°F (200°C).
2. Place the pita breads on a baking sheet.
3. Spread the mashed avocado evenly over each pita bread.
4. Create a small well in the center of each avocado-covered pita and crack an egg into each well.
5. Scatter the cherry tomatoes and crumbled feta cheese over the top.
6. Drizzle with olive oil and season with salt and pepper.
7. Bake in the preheated oven for 10-12 minutes, or until the eggs are cooked to your liking.
8. Remove from the oven and garnish with fresh basil leaves.
9. Serve immediately.

Nutrition Info (per serving)

- Calories: 320
- Protein: 13g
- Carbohydrates: 30g
- Fat: 18g
- Fiber: 8g
- Sugars: 2g
- Sodium: 380mg

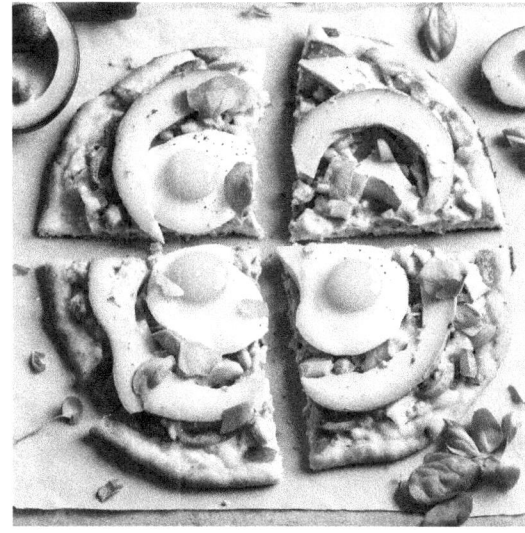

3. Pomegranate and Pistachio Porridge

Servings: 2
Cooking Time: 15 minutes
Ingredients

- 1 cup rolled oats
- 2 cups unsweetened almond milk
- 1/4 cup pomegranate seeds
- 1/4 cup chopped pistachios
- 1 tablespoon honey or maple syrup
- 1/2 teaspoon ground cinnamon
- Pinch of salt

Instructions

1. In a medium saucepan, combine the rolled oats and almond milk.
2. Bring to a simmer over medium heat, stirring occasionally.
3. Cook for about 10 minutes, or until the oats are tender and the porridge has thickened.
4. Stir in the ground cinnamon and a pinch of salt.
5. Divide the porridge between two bowls.
6. Top each bowl with pomegranate seeds, chopped pistachios, and a drizzle of honey or maple syrup.
7. Serve warm.

Nutrition Info (per serving)

- Calories: 350
- Protein: 9g
- Carbohydrates: 50g
- Fat: 13g
- Fiber: 8g
- Sugars: 15g
- Sodium: 150mg

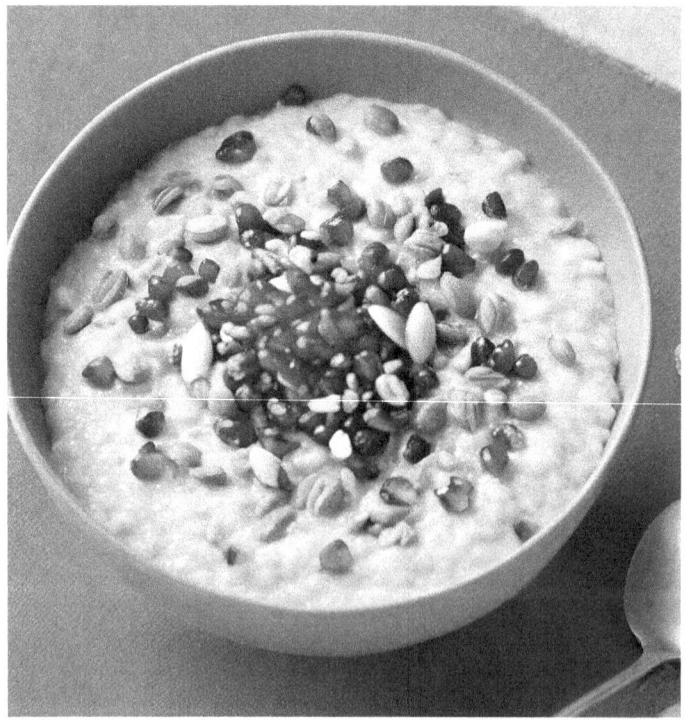

4. Pear and Gorgonzola Salad
Servings: 4
Cooking Time: 10 minutes
Ingredients

- 4 cups mixed greens (such as arugula, spinach, and romaine)
- 2 ripe pears, cored and thinly sliced
- 1/2 cup crumbled Gorgonzola cheese
- 1/4 cup chopped walnuts
- 1/4 cup dried cranberries
- 2 tablespoons olive oil
- 1 tablespoon balsamic vinegar
- Salt and pepper to taste

Instructions

1. In a large bowl, combine the mixed greens, sliced pears, crumbled Gorgonzola cheese, chopped walnuts, and dried cranberries.
2. In a small bowl, whisk together the olive oil and balsamic vinegar. Season with salt and pepper to taste.
3. Drizzle the dressing over the salad and toss gently to combine.
4. Divide the salad among four plates and serve immediately.

Nutrition Info (per serving)

- Calories: 250
- Protein: 5g
- Carbohydrates: 20g
- Fat: 18g
- Fiber: 4g
- Sugars: 12g
- Sodium: 200mg

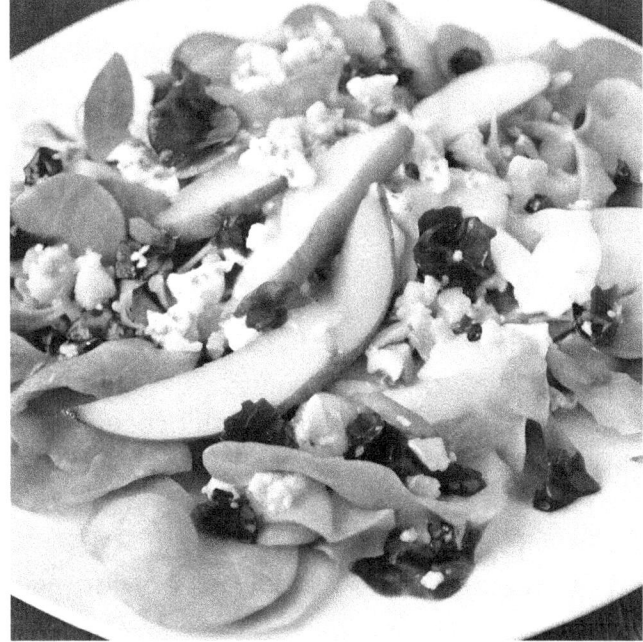

5. Whole Grain Waffles with Blueberry Compote

Servings: 4
Cooking Time: 25 minutes
Ingredients
Waffles:

- 1 1/2 cups whole grain flour
- 2 teaspoons baking powder
- 1/2 teaspoon baking soda
- 1/4 teaspoon ground cinnamon
- 1/4 teaspoon salt
- 1 1/4 cups unsweetened almond milk
- 1 large egg
- 2 tablespoons melted coconut oil
- 1 tablespoon honey or maple syrup
- 1 teaspoon vanilla extract

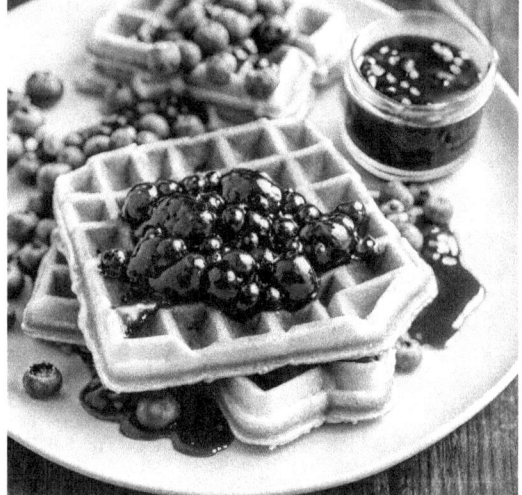

Blueberry Compote:

- 1 cup fresh or frozen blueberries
- 2 tablespoons water
- 1 tablespoon honey or maple syrup
- 1/2 teaspoon lemon zest

Instructions

1. For the Waffles: In a large bowl, whisk together the whole grain flour, baking powder, baking soda, cinnamon, and salt.
2. In a separate bowl, mix the almond milk, egg, melted coconut oil, honey or maple syrup, and vanilla extract.
3. Combine the wet ingredients with the dry ingredients and stir until just combined.
4. Preheat your waffle iron and lightly grease it with coconut oil.
5. Pour the batter into the waffle iron and cook according to the manufacturer's instructions until golden brown and crisp.
6. For the Blueberry Compote: In a small saucepan, combine the blueberries, water, honey or maple syrup, and lemon zest.
7. Cook over medium heat until the blueberries burst and the mixture thickens, about 10 minutes.
8. Serve the waffles warm, topped with the blueberry compote.

Nutrition Info (per serving)

- Calories: 280 Protein: 6g Carbohydrates: 43g   Fat: 10g
- Fiber: 6g
- Sugars: 14g
- Sodium: 300mg

6. Cucumber and Mint Smoothie

Servings: 2

Cooking Time: 10 minutes

Ingredients

- 1 large cucumber, peeled and chopped
- 1 cup unsweetened almond milk
- 1/2 cup Greek yogurt
- 1/4 cup fresh mint leaves
- 1 tablespoon honey or maple syrup
- 1 teaspoon lemon juice
- 1/2 cup ice cubes

Instructions

1. In a blender, combine the cucumber, almond milk, Greek yogurt, mint leaves, honey or maple syrup, lemon juice, and ice cubes.
2. Blend until smooth.
3. Pour into glasses and serve immediately.

Nutrition Info (per serving)

- Calories: 120
- Protein: 5g
- Carbohydrates: 20g
- Fat: 3g
- Fiber: 2g
- Sugars: 14g
- Sodium: 60mg

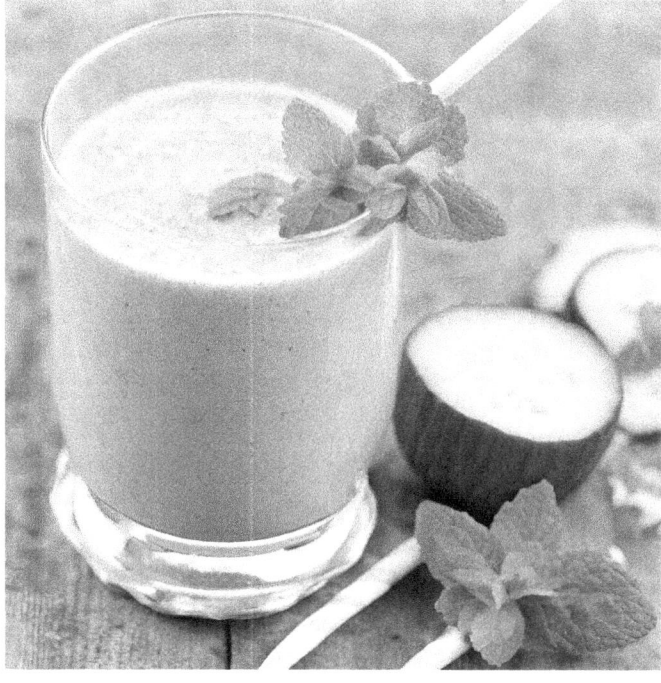

7. Kiwi and Strawberry Salad

Servings: 4
Cooking Time: 10 minutes
Ingredients

- 4 kiwis, peeled and sliced
- 2 cups strawberries, hulled and sliced
- 1 tablespoon fresh lime juice
- 1 tablespoon honey or maple syrup
- 1 tablespoon chopped fresh mint

Instructions

1. In a large bowl, combine the sliced kiwis and strawberries.
2. In a small bowl, whisk together the lime juice and honey or maple syrup.
3. Drizzle the dressing over the fruit and toss gently to combine.
4. Sprinkle with chopped mint and serve immediately.

Nutrition Info (per serving)

- Calories: 90
- Protein: 1g
- Carbohydrates: 23g
- Fat: 0g
- Fiber: 4g
- Sugars: 16g
- Sodium: 10mg

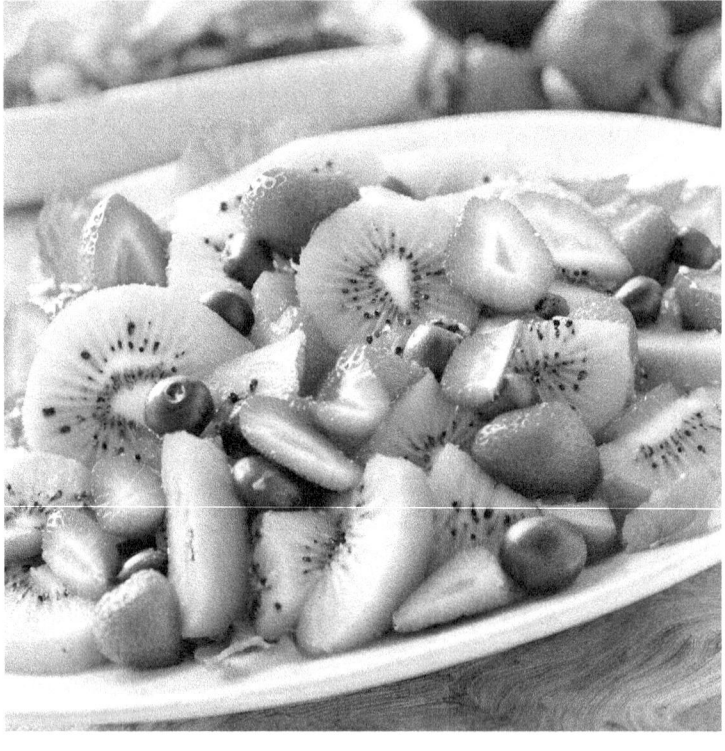

8. Savory Oatmeal with Tomato and Spinach

Servings: 2

Cooking Time: 15 minutes

Ingredients

- 1 cup rolled oats
- 2 cups unsweetened almond milk
- 1 cup fresh spinach, chopped
- 1/2 cup cherry tomatoes, halved
- 1/4 teaspoon ground turmeric
- 1/4 teaspoon paprika
- 1/4 teaspoon garlic powder
- 1 tablespoon nutritional yeast (optional)
- Fresh herbs (basil, parsley) for garnish

Instructions

1. In a medium saucepan, combine the rolled oats and almond milk. Bring to a simmer over medium heat, stirring occasionally.
2. Cook for about 10 minutes, until the oats are tender and the mixture has thickened.
3. Stir in the spinach, cherry tomatoes, turmeric, paprika, garlic powder, and nutritional yeast, if using.
4. Cook for an additional 2-3 minutes, until the spinach is wilted and the tomatoes are softened.
5. Divide the oatmeal between two bowls and garnish with fresh herbs.
6. Serve immediately.

Nutrition Info (per serving)

- Calories: 250
- Protein: 10g
- Carbohydrates: 40g
- Fat: 6g
- Fiber: 7g
- Sugars: 7g
- Sodium: 150mg

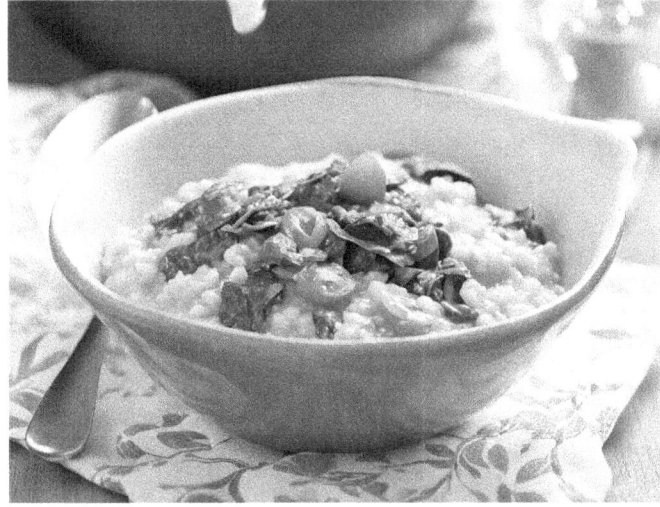

9. Egg and Quinoa Breakfast Cups

Servings: 6
Cooking Time: 25 minutes

Ingredients

- 1 cup cooked quinoa
- 6 large eggs
- 1/2 cup chopped fresh spinach
- 1/2 cup cherry tomatoes, chopped
- 1/4 cup crumbled feta cheese
- 1/4 teaspoon ground black pepper
- 1/4 teaspoon paprika
- Fresh herbs (parsley, chives) for garnish

Instructions

1. Preheat your oven to 350°F (175°C). Lightly grease a muffin tin with coconut oil or cooking spray.
2. In a large bowl, whisk the eggs. Stir in the cooked quinoa, spinach, cherry tomatoes, feta cheese, black pepper, and paprika.
3. Pour the mixture evenly into the prepared muffin tin.
4. Bake for 20-25 minutes, until the eggs are set and the tops are golden brown.
5. Let the breakfast cups cool for a few minutes before removing them from the tin.
6. Garnish with fresh herbs and serve warm.

Nutrition Info (per serving)

- Calories: 150
- Protein: 10g
- Carbohydrates: 12g
- Fat: 7g
- Fiber: 2g
- Sugars: 1g
- Sodium: 120mg

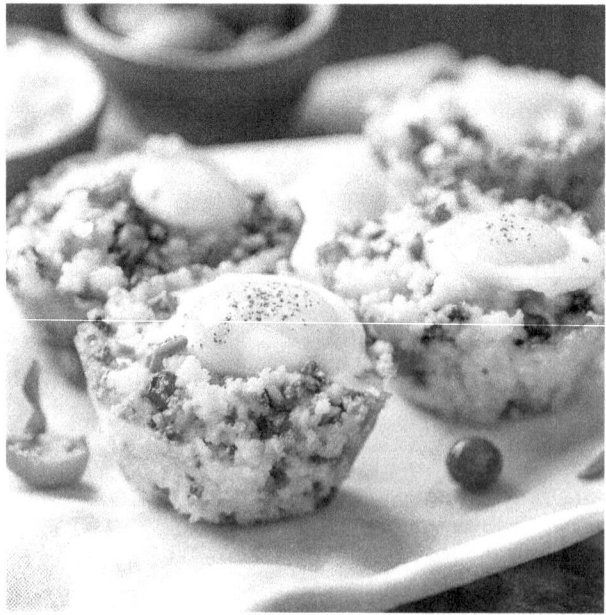

10. Zucchini Bread
Servings: 10 slices
Cooking Time: 1 hour
Ingredients

- 1 1/2 cups whole grain flour
- 1 teaspoon baking powder
- 1/2 teaspoon baking soda
- 1 teaspoon ground cinnamon
- 1/4 teaspoon ground nutmeg
- 1/4 teaspoon salt
- 1 cup grated zucchini
- 1/2 cup unsweetened applesauce
- 1/4 cup honey or maple syrup
- 2 large eggs
- 1/4 cup melted coconut oil
- 1 teaspoon vanilla extract
- 1/4 cup chopped walnuts (optional)

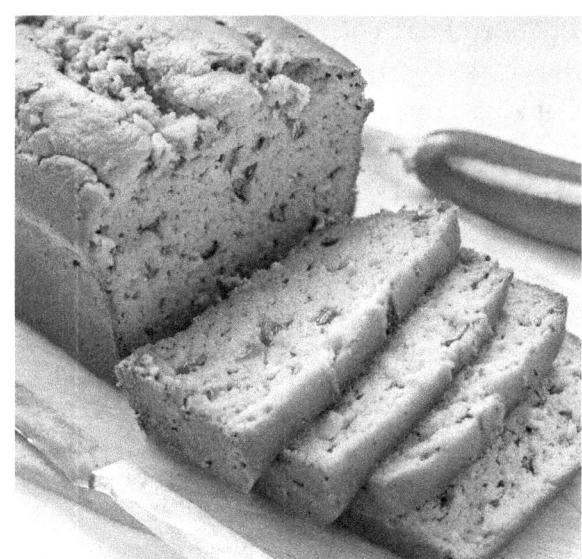

Instructions

1. Preheat your oven to 350°F (175°C). Lightly grease a loaf pan with coconut oil or cooking spray.
2. In a large bowl, whisk together the whole grain flour, baking powder, baking soda, cinnamon, nutmeg, and salt.
3. In a separate bowl, mix the grated zucchini, applesauce, honey or maple syrup, eggs, melted coconut oil, and vanilla extract.
4. Combine the wet ingredients with the dry ingredients and stir until just combined. Fold in the chopped walnuts, if using.
5. Pour the batter into the prepared loaf pan and smooth the top.
6. Bake for 45-50 minutes, or until a toothpick inserted into the center comes out clean.
7. Let the bread cool in the pan for 10 minutes, then transfer to a wire rack to cool completely.
8. Slice and serve.

Nutrition Info (per slice)

- Calories: 180
- Protein: 4g
- Carbohydrates: 26g
- Fat: 7g
- Fiber: 3g
- Sugars: 10g
- Sodium: 180mg

11. Baked Pear with Honey and Walnuts

Servings: 4

Cooking Time: 30 minutes

Ingredients

- 4 ripe pears, halved and cored
- 2 tablespoons honey
- 1/4 cup chopped walnuts
- 1 teaspoon ground cinnamon
- 1/4 teaspoon ground nutmeg

Instructions

1. Preheat your oven to 350°F (175°C).
2. Place the pear halves cut side up in a baking dish.
3. Drizzle each pear half with honey.
4. Sprinkle the chopped walnuts evenly over the pears.
5. Dust the pears with ground cinnamon and nutmeg.
6. Bake in the preheated oven for 25-30 minutes, until the pears are tender.
7. Serve warm.

Nutrition Info (per serving)

- Calories: 180
- Protein: 2g
- Carbohydrates: 32g
- Fat: 6g
- Fiber: 5g
- Sugars: 24g
- Sodium: 0mg

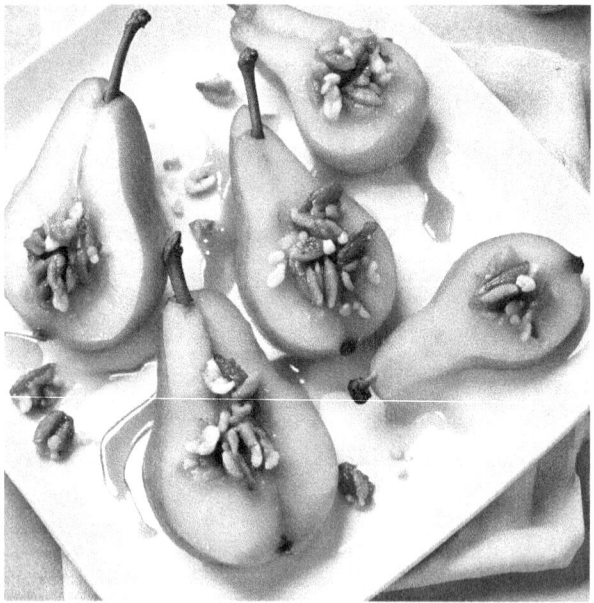

12. Spinach and Avocado Wrap

Servings: 2
Cooking Time: 10 minutes
Ingredients

- 2 whole grain tortillas
- 1 cup fresh spinach leaves
- 1 ripe avocado, sliced
- 1/4 cup crumbled feta cheese
- 1/2 cup cherry tomatoes, halved
- 1 tablespoon hummus
- 1 teaspoon lemon juice
- Fresh herbs (parsley, cilantro) for garnish

Instructions

1. Lay the tortillas flat on a clean surface.
2. Spread the hummus evenly over each tortilla.
3. Layer the spinach leaves, avocado slices, crumbled feta cheese, and cherry tomatoes on each tortilla.
4. Drizzle with lemon juice.
5. Sprinkle fresh herbs over the top.
6. Roll up the tortillas tightly, tucking in the sides as you go.
7. Slice in half and serve immediately.

Nutrition Info (per serving)

- Calories: 320
- Protein: 9g
- Carbohydrates: 40g
- Fat: 16g
- Fiber: 10g
- Sugars: 3g
- Sodium: 260mg

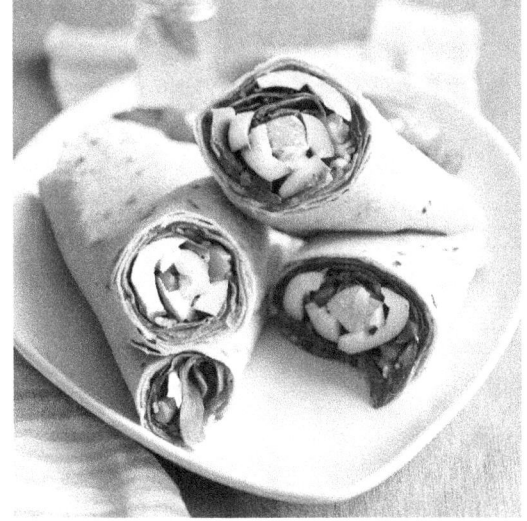

13. Walnut and Banana Smoothie

Servings: 2
Cooking Time: 5 minutes
Ingredients

- 1 ripe banana
- 1/4 cup walnuts
- 1 cup unsweetened almond milk
- 1/2 cup Greek yogurt
- 1 tablespoon honey or maple syrup
- 1/2 teaspoon ground cinnamon
- 1/2 cup ice cubes

Instructions

1. In a blender, combine the banana, walnuts, almond milk, Greek yogurt, honey or maple syrup, ground cinnamon, and ice cubes.
2. Blend until smooth.
3. Pour into glasses and serve immediately.

Nutrition Info (per serving)

- Calories: 250
- Protein: 8g
- Carbohydrates: 32g
- Fat: 11g
- Fiber: 4g
- Sugars: 18g
- Sodium: 60mg

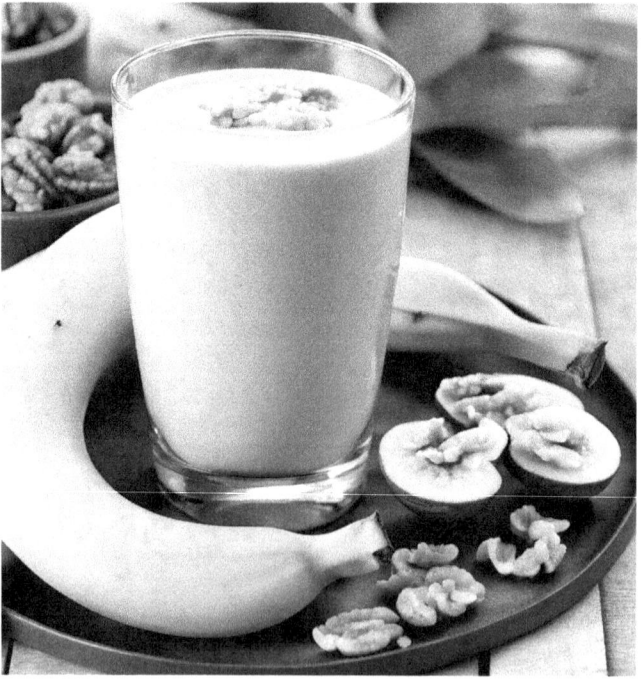

14. Overnight Oats with Mango

Servings: 2

Cooking Time: 10 minutes (plus overnight refrigeration)

Ingredients

- 1 cup rolled oats
- 1 cup unsweetened almond milk
- 1/2 cup Greek yogurt
- 1 ripe mango, diced
- 1 tablespoon chia seeds
- 1 tablespoon honey or maple syrup
- 1/2 teaspoon vanilla extract

Instructions

1. In a medium bowl, combine the rolled oats, almond milk, Greek yogurt, chia seeds, honey or maple syrup, and vanilla extract.
2. Stir well to combine.
3. Divide the mixture into two jars or bowls.
4. Top each with diced mango.
5. Cover and refrigerate overnight.
6. Serve chilled in the morning.

Nutrition Info (per serving)

- Calories: 350
- Protein: 11g
- Carbohydrates: 61g
- Fat: 8g
- Fiber: 10g
- Sugars: 24g
- Sodium: 90mg

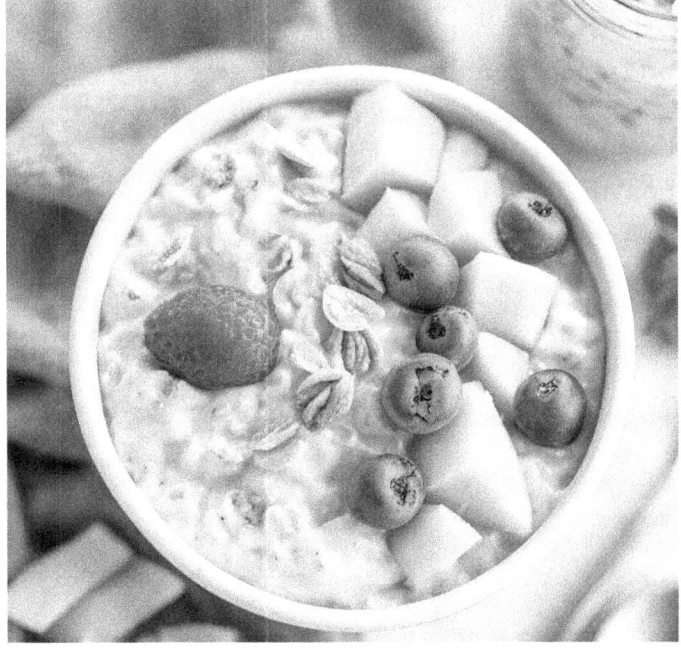

15. Tofu Scramble

Servings: 2
Cooking Time: 15 minutes
Ingredients

- 1 block (14 oz) firm tofu, drained and crumbled
- 1 tablespoon olive oil
- 1/2 cup chopped onion
- 1/2 cup chopped bell pepper
- 1 cup fresh spinach, chopped
- 1/2 teaspoon ground turmeric
- 1/4 teaspoon garlic powder
- 1/4 teaspoon paprika
- Fresh herbs (parsley, chives) for garnish

Instructions

1. Heat the olive oil in a large skillet over medium heat.
2. Add the chopped onion and bell pepper and sauté until softened, about 5 minutes.
3. Add the crumbled tofu, ground turmeric, garlic powder, and paprika to the skillet. Stir to combine.
4. Cook for about 5-7 minutes, stirring occasionally, until the tofu is heated through and slightly golden.
5. Add the chopped spinach and cook until wilted, about 2 minutes.
6. Garnish with fresh herbs and serve immediately.

Nutrition Info (per serving)

- Calories: 200
- Protein: 14g
- Carbohydrates: 10g
- Fat: 12g
- Fiber: 4g
- Sugars: 2g
- Sodium: 200mg

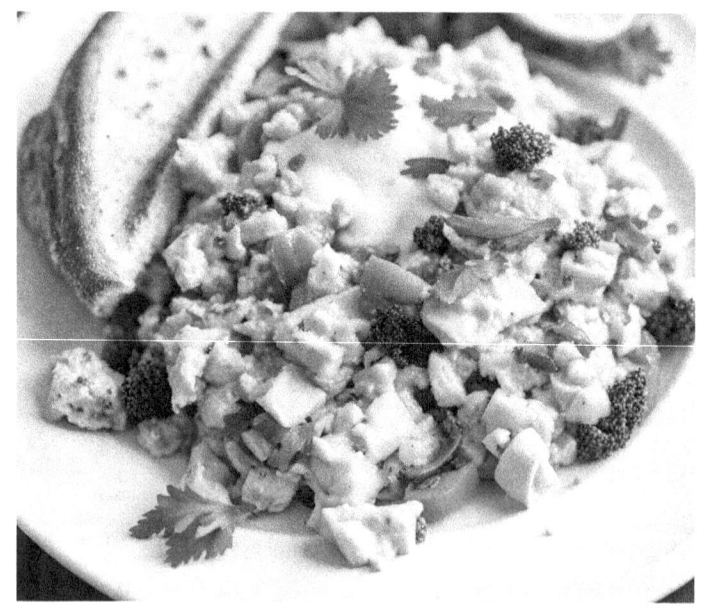

16. Apple Cinnamon Porridge

Servings: 2
Cooking Time: 15 minutes

Ingredients

- 1 cup rolled oats
- 2 cups unsweetened almond milk
- 1 apple, peeled, cored, and diced
- 1 tablespoon honey or maple syrup
- 1 teaspoon ground cinnamon
- 1/4 teaspoon ground nutmeg
- 1/4 cup chopped walnuts

Instructions

1. In a medium saucepan, combine the rolled oats, almond milk, diced apple, honey or maple syrup, ground cinnamon, and ground nutmeg.
2. Bring to a simmer over medium heat, stirring occasionally.
3. Cook for about 10-15 minutes, until the oats are tender and the porridge has thickened.
4. Divide the porridge between two bowls.
5. Top each bowl with chopped walnuts.
6. Serve warm.

Nutrition Info (per serving)

- Calories: 300
- Protein: 7g
- Carbohydrates: 50g
- Fat: 10g
- Fiber: 7g
- Sugars: 20g
- Sodium: 90mg

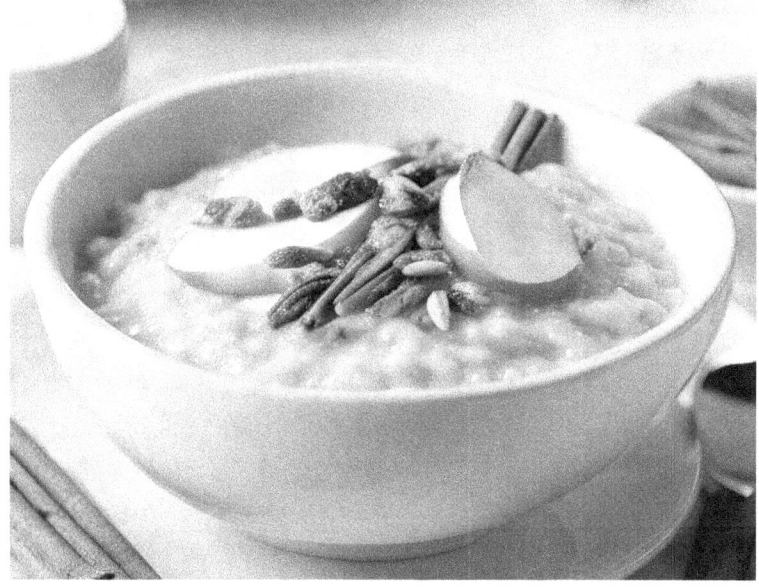

18. Broccoli and Cheese Oatmeal

Servings: 2
Cooking Time: 20 minutes
Ingredients

- 1 cup rolled oats
- 2 cups unsweetened almond milk
- 1 cup small broccoli florets
- 1/2 cup grated cheddar cheese
- 1/2 teaspoon garlic powder
- 1/4 teaspoon paprika
- Fresh herbs (chives, parsley) for garnish

Instructions

1. In a medium saucepan, bring the almond milk to a simmer over medium heat.
2. Add the rolled oats and cook for about 5 minutes, stirring occasionally.
3. Add the broccoli florets and cook for an additional 5-7 minutes, until the oats are tender and the broccoli is cooked.
4. Stir in the grated cheddar cheese, garlic powder, and paprika.
5. Cook for another 2-3 minutes, until the cheese is melted and well combined.
6. Divide the oatmeal between two bowls and garnish with fresh herbs.
7. Serve warm.

Nutrition Info (per serving)

- Calories: 350
- Protein: 15g
- Carbohydrates: 45g
- Fat: 15g
- Fiber: 7g
- Sugars: 6g
- Sodium: 220mg

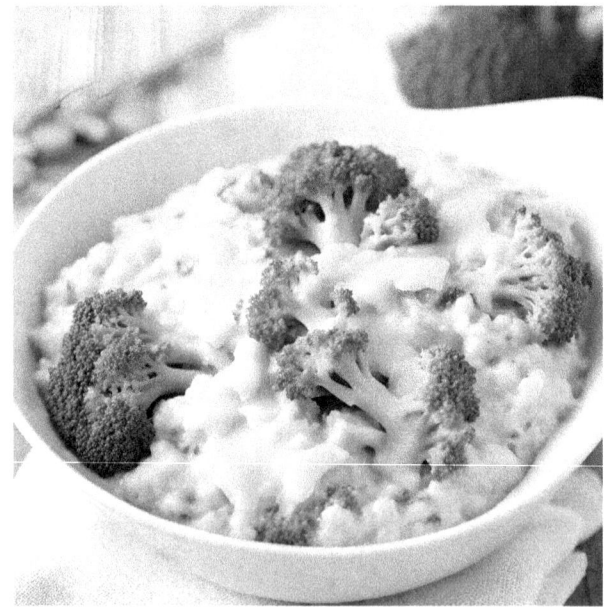

19. Peach and Raspberry Smoothie
Servings: 2
Cooking Time: 5 minutes
Ingredients

- 2 ripe peaches, pitted and sliced
- 1 cup fresh or frozen raspberries
- 1 cup unsweetened almond milk
- 1/2 cup Greek yogurt
- 1 tablespoon honey or maple syrup
- 1/2 cup ice cubes

Instructions

1. In a blender, combine the peaches, raspberries, almond milk, Greek yogurt, honey or maple syrup, and ice cubes.
2. Blend until smooth.
3. Pour into glasses and serve immediately.

Nutrition Info (per serving)

- Calories: 200
- Protein: 6g
- Carbohydrates: 38g
- Fat: 4g
- Fiber: 6g
- Sugars: 27g
- Sodium: 50mg

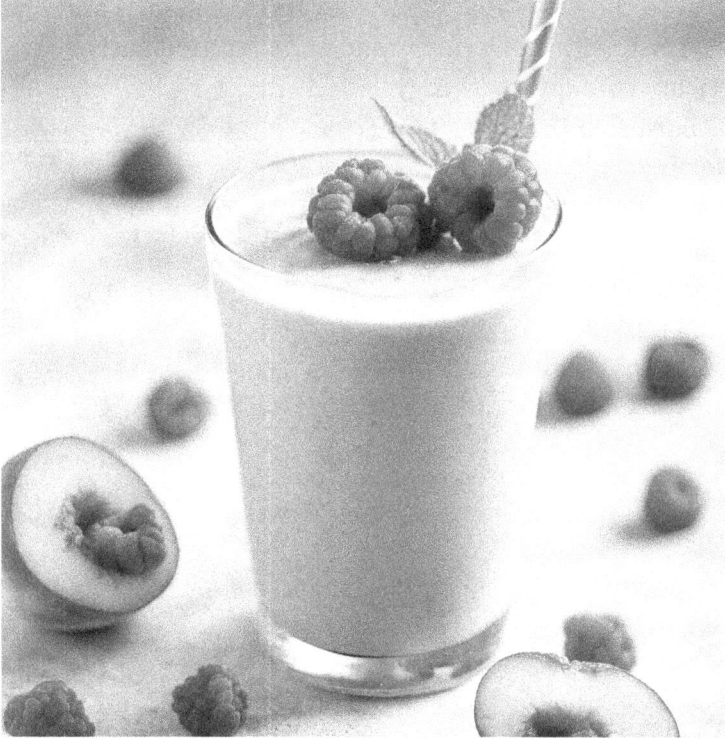

20. Vegetable Hash with Poached Egg

Servings: 2
Cooking Time: 30 minutes
Ingredients

- 1 tablespoon olive oil
- 1 small onion, chopped
- 1 red bell pepper, chopped
- 1 zucchini, chopped
- 1 cup sweet potato, peeled and diced
- 1/2 teaspoon ground turmeric
- 1/4 teaspoon ground cumin
- 2 large eggs
- Fresh herbs (cilantro, parsley) for garnish

Instructions

1. Heat the olive oil in a large skillet over medium heat.
2. Add the chopped onion, red bell pepper, zucchini, and sweet potato. Cook for about 10-15 minutes, until the vegetables are tender.
3. Stir in the ground turmeric and cumin. Cook for another 2-3 minutes.
4. In a separate pot, bring water to a simmer and poach the eggs for about 3-4 minutes, until the whites are set and the yolks are runny.
5. Divide the vegetable hash between two plates and top each with a poached egg.
6. Garnish with fresh herbs and serve immediately.

Nutrition Info (per serving)

- Calories: 300
- Protein: 10g
- Carbohydrates: 35g
- Fat: 14g
- Fiber: 8g
- Sugars: 10g
- Sodium: 90mg

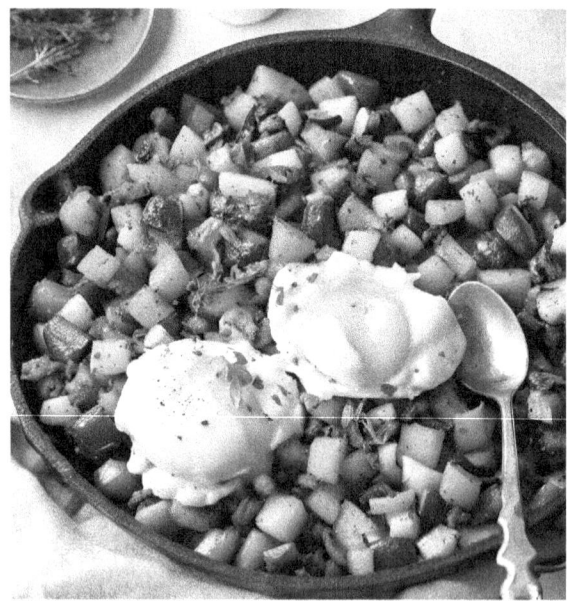

21. Almond Butter and Banana Sandwich

Servings: 2

Cooking Time: 5 minutes

Ingredients

- 4 slices whole grain bread
- 4 tablespoons almond butter
- 2 bananas, sliced
- 1 tablespoon honey (optional)

Instructions

1. Toast the slices of whole grain bread if desired.
2. Spread 2 tablespoons of almond butter on each of two slices of bread.
3. Layer the banana slices evenly over the almond butter.
4. Drizzle with honey if using.
5. Top with the remaining slices of bread to make sandwiches.
6. Serve immediately.

Nutrition Info (per serving)

- Calories: 350
- Protein: 10g
- Carbohydrates: 55g
- Fat: 12g
- Fiber: 8g
- Sugars: 18g
- Sodium: 180mg

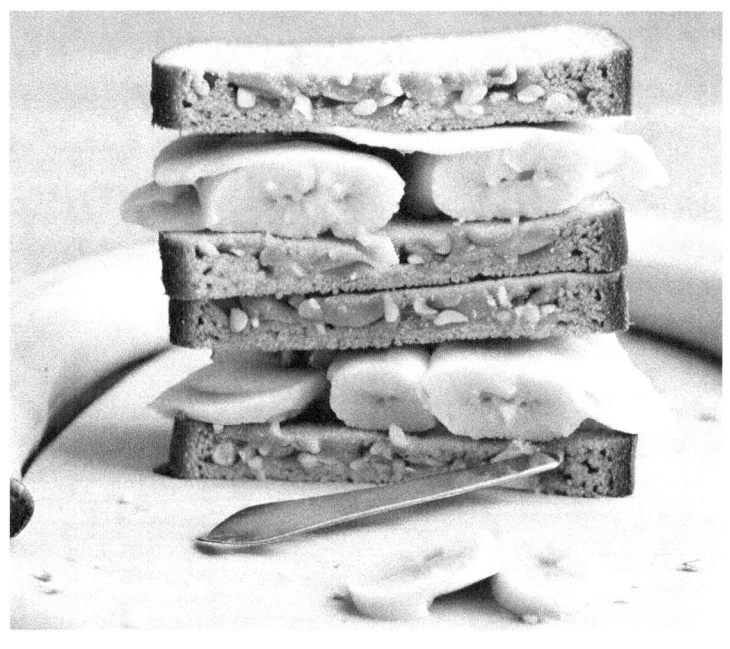

22. Pumpkin Oatmeal

Servings: 2
Cooking Time: 15 minutes
Ingredients

- 1 cup rolled oats
- 2 cups unsweetened almond milk
- 1/2 cup pumpkin puree
- 1 tablespoon honey or maple syrup
- 1 teaspoon ground cinnamon
- 1/4 teaspoon ground nutmeg
- 1/4 teaspoon ground ginger
- 1/4 cup chopped pecans

Instructions

1. In a medium saucepan, combine the rolled oats, almond milk, pumpkin puree, honey or maple syrup, ground cinnamon, nutmeg, and ginger.
2. Bring to a simmer over medium heat, stirring occasionally.
3. Cook for about 10-15 minutes, until the oats are tender and the mixture has thickened.
4. Divide the oatmeal between two bowls.
5. Top each bowl with chopped pecans.
6. Serve warm.

Nutrition Info (per serving)

- Calories: 280
- Protein: 6g
- Carbohydrates: 45g
- Fat: 10g
- Fiber: 7g
- Sugars: 18g
- Sodium: 80mg

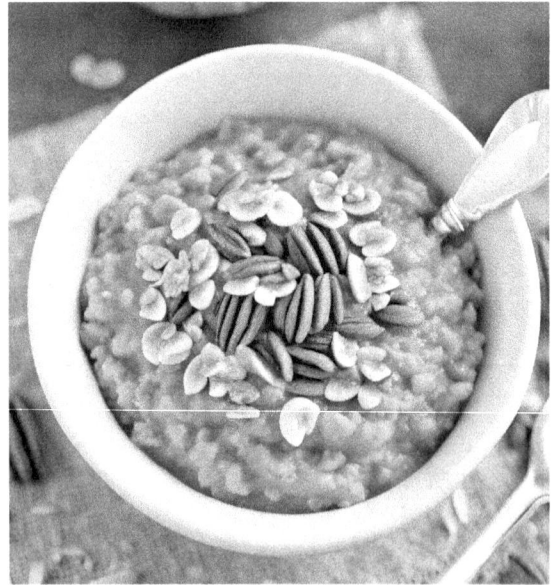

23. Greek Yogurt Parfait

Servings: 2
Cooking Time: 5 minutes

Ingredients

- 2 cups Greek yogurt
- 1 cup mixed berries (strawberries, blueberries, raspberries)
- 1/4 cup granola (low sugar)
- 1 tablespoon honey or maple syrup
- 1 tablespoon chia seeds

Instructions

1. In two serving glasses, layer half of the Greek yogurt.
2. Add a layer of mixed berries.
3. Sprinkle with granola.
4. Repeat the layers with the remaining Greek yogurt, berries, and granola.
5. Drizzle with honey or maple syrup.
6. Top with chia seeds.
7. Serve immediately.

Nutrition Info (per serving)

- Calories: 250
- Protein: 20g
- Carbohydrates: 32g
- Fat: 6g
- Fiber: 5g
- Sugars: 20g
- Sodium: 60mg

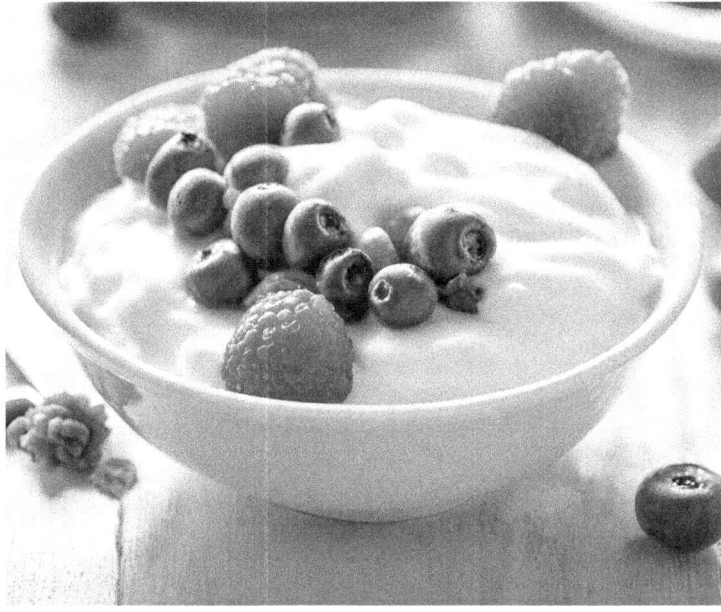

24. Mushroom and Spinach Toast

Servings: 2

Cooking Time: 15 minutes

Ingredients

- 4 slices whole grain bread
- 1 tablespoon olive oil
- 1 cup mushrooms, sliced
- 1 cup fresh spinach leaves
- 1/2 teaspoon garlic powder
- 1/2 teaspoon ground paprika
- 1/4 cup crumbled feta cheese
- Fresh herbs (parsley, thyme) for garnish

Instructions

1. Toast the whole grain bread slices.
2. Heat the olive oil in a skillet over medium heat.
3. Add the mushrooms and cook for about 5 minutes until they are tender.
4. Add the spinach, garlic powder, and paprika. Cook for an additional 2-3 minutes until the spinach is wilted.
5. Top the toasted bread with the mushroom and spinach mixture.
6. Sprinkle with crumbled feta cheese and garnish with fresh herbs.
7. Serve immediately.

Nutrition Info (per serving)

- Calories: 240
- Protein: 8g
- Carbohydrates: 28g
- Fat: 12g
- Fiber: 6g
- Sugars: 4g
- Sodium: 220mg

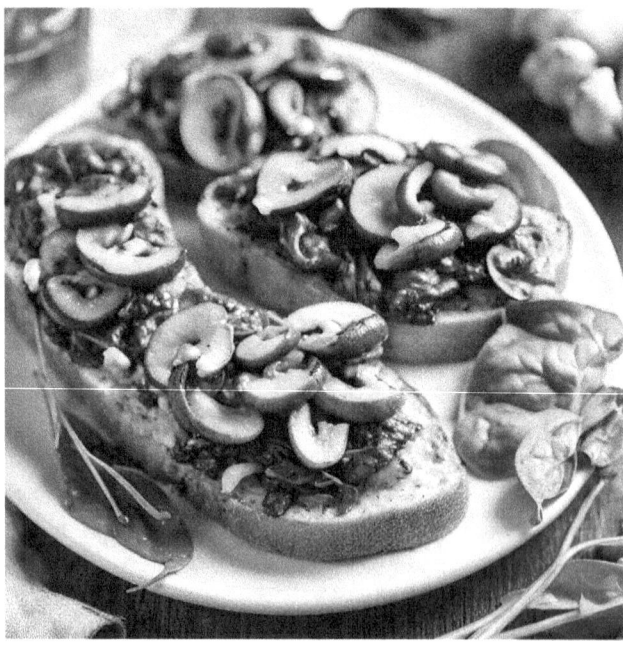

25. Banana Pancakes
Servings: 4
Cooking Time: 20 minutes
Ingredients
- 1 cup whole grain flour
- 1 tablespoon baking powder
- 1 teaspoon ground cinnamon
- 1/4 teaspoon ground nutmeg
- 1 cup unsweetened almond milk
- 1 large ripe banana, mashed
- 1 tablespoon honey or maple syrup
- 1 teaspoon vanilla extract
- 1 tablespoon coconut oil, melted

Instructions
1. In a large bowl, whisk together the whole grain flour, baking powder, ground cinnamon, and nutmeg.
2. In another bowl, combine the almond milk, mashed banana, honey or maple syrup, vanilla extract, and melted coconut oil.
3. Pour the wet ingredients into the dry ingredients and stir until just combined.
4. Heat a non-stick skillet over medium heat and lightly grease with coconut oil.
5. Pour 1/4 cup of batter onto the skillet for each pancake.
6. Cook for about 2-3 minutes until bubbles form on the surface, then flip and cook for another 2-3 minutes until golden brown.
7. Repeat with the remaining batter.
8. Serve warm.

Nutrition Info (per serving)
- Calories: 200
- Protein: 4g
- Carbohydrates: 35g
- Fat: 6g
- Fiber: 4g
- Sugars: 9g
- Sodium: 180mg

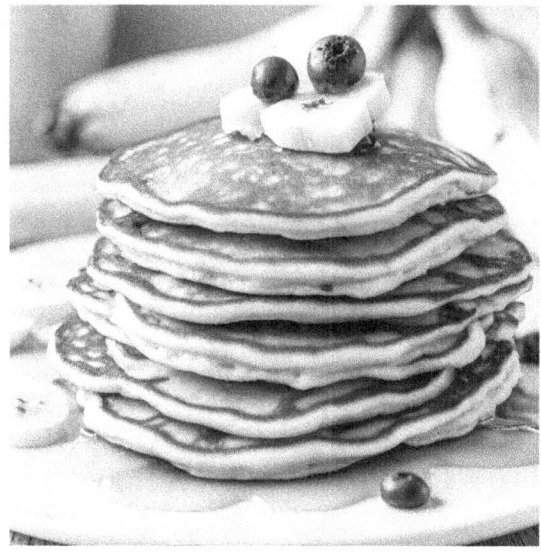

26. Cottage Cheese with Pineapple and Chia Seeds

Servings: 2

Cooking Time: 5 minutes

Ingredients

- 2 cups low-fat cottage cheese
- 1 cup fresh pineapple chunks
- 2 tablespoons chia seeds
- 1 tablespoon honey or maple syrup

Instructions

1. Divide the cottage cheese between two bowls.
2. Top each bowl with fresh pineapple chunks.
3. Sprinkle with chia seeds.
4. Drizzle with honey or maple syrup.
5. Serve immediately.

Nutrition Info (per serving)

- Calories: 220
- Protein: 20g
- Carbohydrates: 22g
- Fat: 6g
- Fiber: 4g
- Sugars: 18g
- Sodium: 360mg

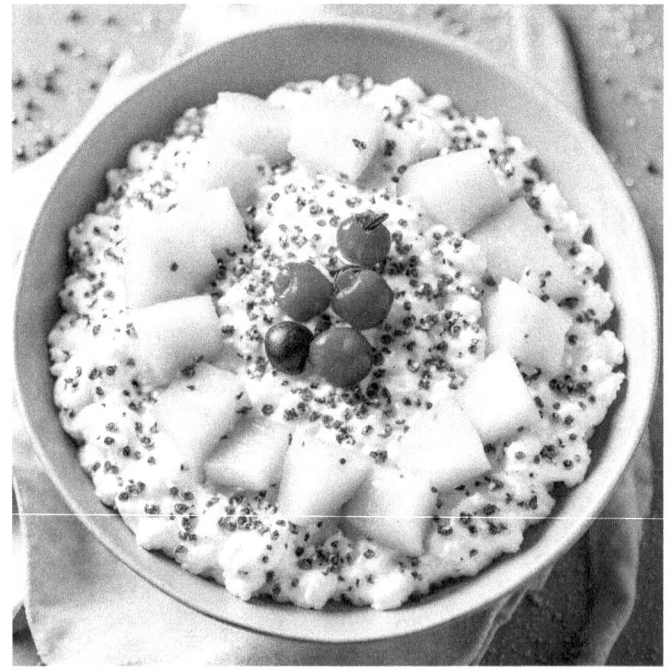

27. Sweet Potato and Black Bean Burrito
Servings: 2
Cooking Time: 30 minutes
Ingredients
- 1 medium sweet potato, peeled and diced
- 1 tablespoon olive oil
- 1/2 teaspoon ground cumin
- 1/2 teaspoon ground paprika
- 1 cup canned black beans, rinsed and drained
- 1/2 cup fresh salsa
- 2 whole grain tortillas
- 1/4 cup chopped fresh cilantro

Instructions
1. Preheat the oven to 400°F (200°C).
2. Toss the diced sweet potato with olive oil, ground cumin, and paprika.
3. Spread the sweet potato on a baking sheet and roast for 20 minutes until tender.
4. In a skillet, heat the black beans until warm.
5. Assemble the burritos by placing roasted sweet potato, black beans, and salsa on each tortilla.
6. Roll up the tortillas and top with fresh cilantro.
7. Serve immediately.

Nutrition Info (per serving)
- Calories: 350
- Protein: 10g
- Carbohydrates: 60g
- Fat: 9g
- Fiber: 12g
- Sugars: 9g
- Sodium: 400mg

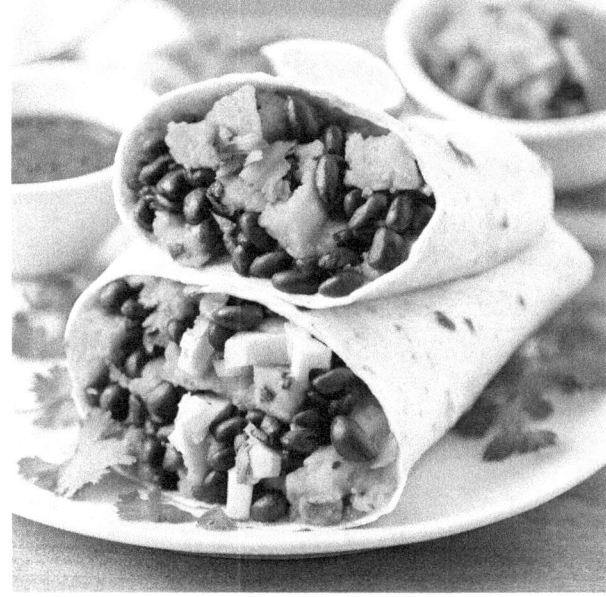

28. Oatmeal with Mixed Nuts and Berries

Servings: 2
Cooking Time: 15 minutes
Ingredients

- 1 cup rolled oats
- 2 cups unsweetened almond milk
- 1/4 cup mixed nuts (almonds, walnuts, pecans), chopped
- 1/2 cup mixed berries (blueberries, strawberries, raspberries)
- 1 tablespoon honey or maple syrup
- 1/2 teaspoon ground cinnamon

Instructions

1. In a medium saucepan, combine the rolled oats and almond milk. Bring to a simmer over medium heat, stirring occasionally.
2. Cook for about 10 minutes, until the oats are tender and the mixture has thickened.
3. Divide the oatmeal between two bowls.
4. Top each bowl with mixed nuts, berries, honey or maple syrup, and ground cinnamon.
5. Serve warm.

Nutrition Info (per serving)

- Calories: 300
- Protein: 8g
- Carbohydrates: 45g
- Fat: 10g
- Fiber: 8g
- Sugars: 15g
- Sodium: 50mg

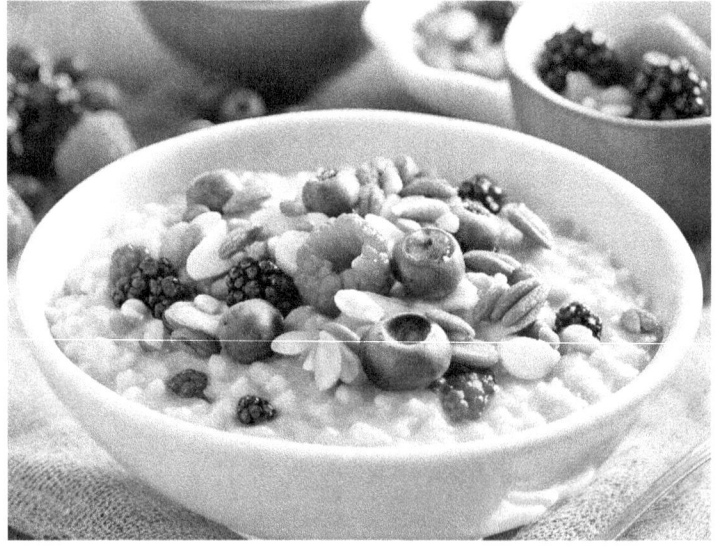

29. Carrot and Apple Muffins

Servings: 12 muffins
Cooking Time: 25 minutes

Ingredients

- 1 1/2 cups whole grain flour
- 1 teaspoon baking powder
- 1/2 teaspoon baking soda
- 1 teaspoon ground cinnamon
- 1/4 teaspoon ground nutmeg
- 1/4 teaspoon ground ginger
- 1/2 teaspoon salt
- 1 cup grated carrots
- 1 cup grated apple
- 2 large eggs
- 1/2 cup unsweetened applesauce
- 1/4 cup honey or maple syrup
- 1/4 cup melted coconut oil
- 1 teaspoon vanilla extract

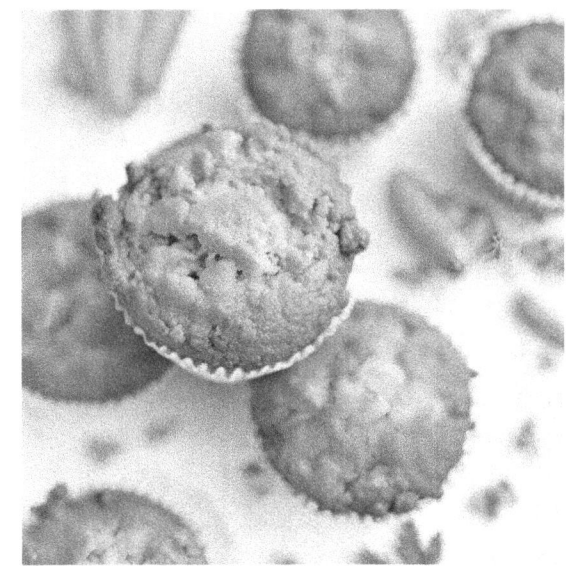

Instructions

1. Preheat the oven to 350°F (175°C). Line a muffin tin with paper liners.
2. In a large bowl, whisk together the whole grain flour, baking powder, baking soda, ground cinnamon, nutmeg, ginger, and salt.
3. In another bowl, mix the grated carrots, grated apple, eggs, applesauce, honey or maple syrup, melted coconut oil, and vanilla extract.
4. Pour the wet ingredients into the dry ingredients and stir until just combined.
5. Divide the batter evenly among the muffin cups.
6. Bake for 20-25 minutes, until a toothpick inserted into the center comes out clean.
7. Allow to cool in the tin for 5 minutes, then transfer to a wire rack to cool completely.
8. Serve warm or at room temperature.

Nutrition Info (per muffin)

- Calories: 150
- Protein: 3g
- Carbohydrates: 25g
- Fat: 5g
- Fiber: 3g
- Sugars: 12g
- Sodium: 120mg

Fish and Seafood Recipes

1. Grilled Salmon with Avocado Salsa
Servings: 4
Cooking Time: 20 minutes
Ingredients
Salmon:

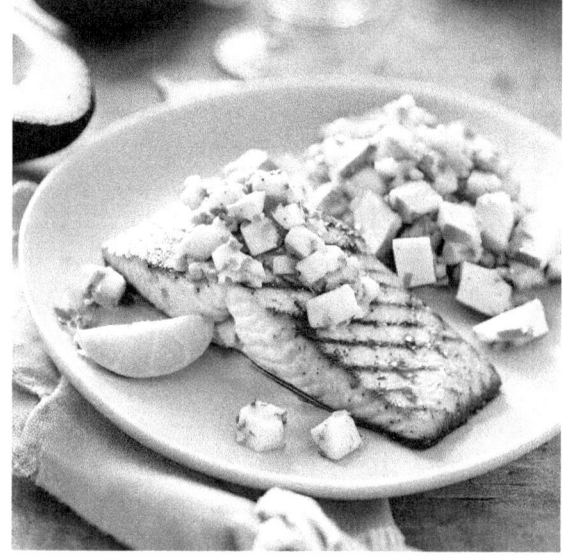

- 4 salmon fillets (6 ounces each)
- 1 tablespoon olive oil
- 1 teaspoon ground cumin
- 1 teaspoon paprika
- 1/2 teaspoon garlic powder
- 1/2 teaspoon onion powder
- 1/2 teaspoon dried oregano
- 1 tablespoon lemon juice

Avocado Salsa:

- 2 ripe avocados, diced
- 1 cup cherry tomatoes, quartered
- 1/4 cup red onion, finely chopped
- 1/4 cup fresh cilantro, chopped
- 1 tablespoon lime juice

Instructions

1. For the Salmon: Preheat the grill to medium-high heat.
2. In a small bowl, mix the olive oil, ground cumin, paprika, garlic powder, onion powder, dried oregano, and lemon juice.
3. Brush the salmon fillets with the seasoning mixture.
4. Grill the salmon for about 4-5 minutes per side, or until the salmon is cooked through and flakes easily with a fork.
5. For the Avocado Salsa: In a medium bowl, combine the diced avocados, cherry tomatoes, red onion, cilantro, and lime juice. Mix gently.
6. Serve the grilled salmon topped with the avocado salsa.

Nutrition Info (per serving)

- Calories: 450 Protein: 35g Carbohydrates: 12g   Fat: 28g
- Fiber: 8g
- Sugars: 2g
- Sodium: 70mg

2. Lemon Herb Baked Cod

Servings: 4
Cooking Time: 25 minutes
Ingredients

- 4 cod fillets (6 ounces each)
- 2 tablespoons olive oil
- 1 tablespoon lemon juice
- 1 teaspoon lemon zest
- 1 teaspoon dried oregano
- 1 teaspoon dried thyme
- 2 garlic cloves, minced
- 1/4 teaspoon paprika
- Fresh parsley for garnish

Instructions

1. Preheat the oven to 400°F (200°C).
2. In a small bowl, combine the olive oil, lemon juice, lemon zest, dried oregano, dried thyme, minced garlic, and paprika.
3. Place the cod fillets in a baking dish and brush with the lemon herb mixture.
4. Bake for 15-20 minutes, or until the cod is cooked through and flakes easily with a fork.
5. Garnish with fresh parsley and serve immediately.

Nutrition Info (per serving)

- Calories: 220
- Protein: 32g
- Carbohydrates: 2g
- Fat: 9g
- Fiber: 0g
- Sugars: 0g
- Sodium: 100mg

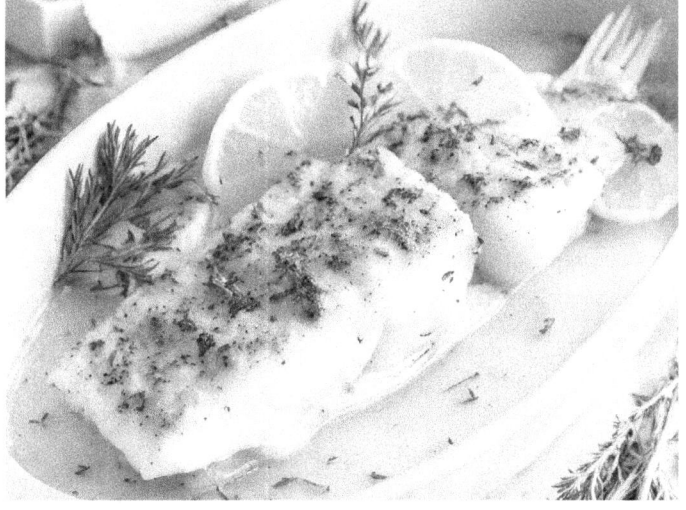

3. Shrimp and Mango Salad

Servings: 4
Cooking Time: 15 minutes
Ingredients

- 1 pound large shrimp, peeled and deveined
- 1 tablespoon olive oil
- 1 mango, peeled and diced
- 1 avocado, diced
- 1 cup cherry tomatoes, halved
- 1/4 cup red onion, finely chopped
- 1/4 cup fresh cilantro, chopped
- 2 tablespoons lime juice
- 1 teaspoon ground cumin

Instructions

1. Heat the olive oil in a large skillet over medium heat.
2. Add the shrimp and cook for about 3-4 minutes on each side, until pink and opaque.
3. In a large bowl, combine the cooked shrimp, diced mango, avocado, cherry tomatoes, red onion, cilantro, lime juice, and ground cumin. Toss gently to combine.
4. Serve immediately.

Nutrition Info (per serving)

- Calories: 280
- Protein: 25g
- Carbohydrates: 18g
- Fat: 14g
- Fiber: 5g
- Sugars: 10g
- Sodium: 300mg

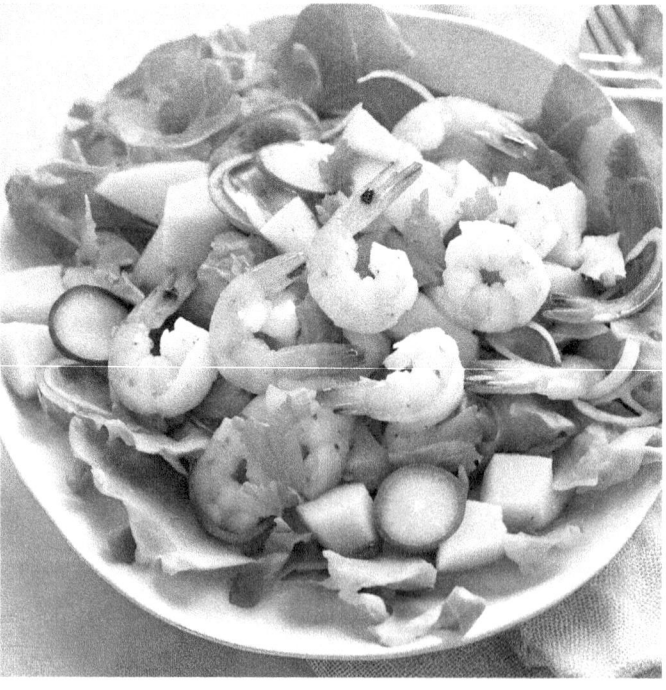

4. Tuna Nicoise Salad
Servings: 4
Cooking Time: 20 minutes
Ingredients

- 2 cans (5 ounces each) tuna in water, drained
- 4 cups mixed greens
- 1 cup green beans, trimmed and blanched
- 1/2 cup cherry tomatoes, halved
- 4 hard-boiled eggs, quartered
- 1/4 cup Kalamata olives, pitted and halved
- 1/4 cup red onion, thinly sliced
- 2 tablespoons olive oil
- 1 tablespoon red wine vinegar
- 1 teaspoon Dijon mustard
- Fresh parsley for garnish

Instructions

1. In a large bowl, arrange the mixed greens, green beans, cherry tomatoes, hard-boiled eggs, Kalamata olives, and red onion.
2. Top with the drained tuna.
3. In a small bowl, whisk together the olive oil, red wine vinegar, and Dijon mustard.
4. Drizzle the dressing over the salad and toss gently to combine.
5. Garnish with fresh parsley and serve immediately.

Nutrition Info (per serving)

- Calories: 300
- Protein: 26g
- Carbohydrates: 10g
- Fat: 18g
- Fiber: 4g
- Sugars: 3g
- Sodium: 350mg

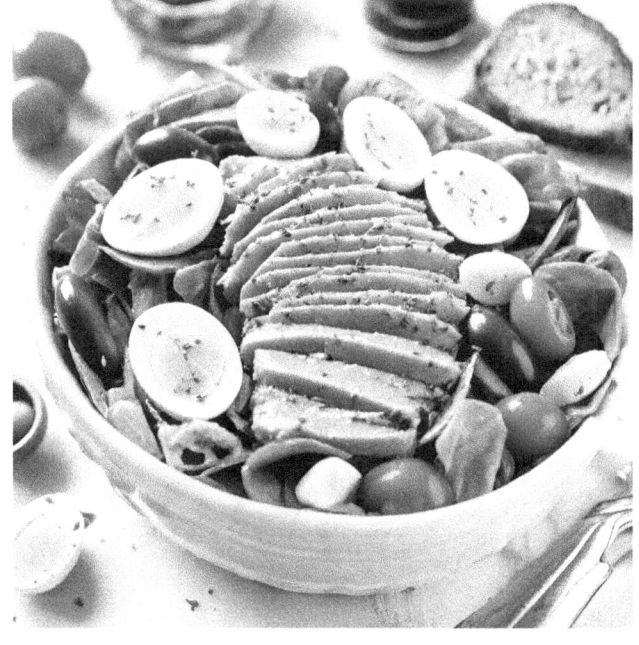

5. Garlic Butter Scallops

Servings: 4
Cooking Time: 15 minutes
Ingredients

- 1 pound large scallops
- 2 tablespoons olive oil
- 3 garlic cloves, minced
- 1/4 cup unsalted butter
- 1 tablespoon lemon juice
- 1 tablespoon chopped fresh parsley

Instructions

1. Pat the scallops dry with paper towels.
2. Heat the olive oil in a large skillet over medium-high heat.
3. Add the scallops and cook for 2-3 minutes on each side until golden brown and opaque.
4. Remove the scallops from the skillet and set aside.
5. In the same skillet, melt the butter over medium heat.
6. Add the minced garlic and cook for 1 minute until fragrant.
7. Stir in the lemon juice and return the scallops to the skillet. Toss to coat in the garlic butter sauce.
8. Garnish with chopped parsley and serve immediately.

Nutrition Info (per serving)

- Calories: 250
- Protein: 20g
- Carbohydrates: 2g
- Fat: 18g
- Fiber: 0g
- Sugars: 0g
- Sodium: 360mg

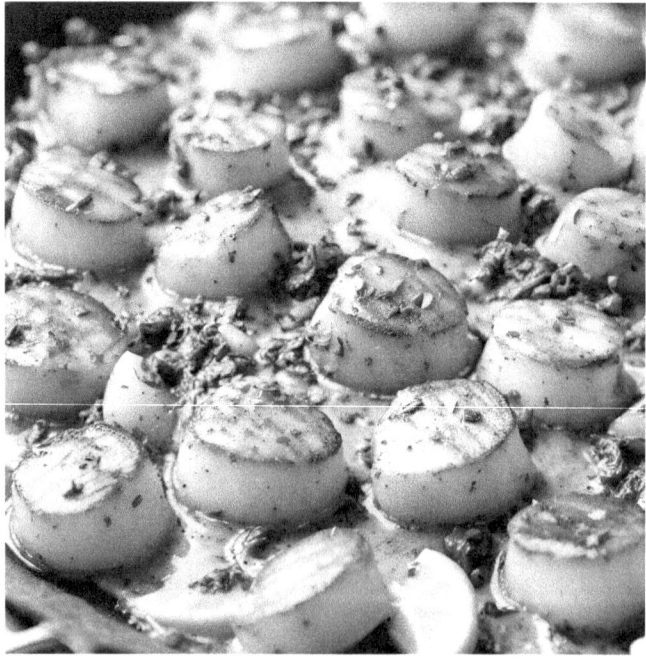

6. Seafood Paella

Servings: 6
Cooking Time: 45 minutes
Ingredients

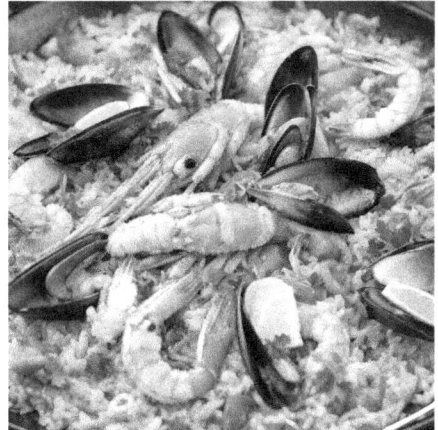

- 1 tablespoon olive oil
- 1 onion, chopped
- 1 red bell pepper, chopped
- 3 garlic cloves, minced
- 1 1/2 cups Arborio rice
- 1 teaspoon smoked paprika
- 1/2 teaspoon ground turmeric
- 4 cups low-sodium chicken or vegetable broth
- 1 cup diced tomatoes
- 1/2 pound shrimp, peeled and deveined
- 1/2 pound mussels, scrubbed and debearded
- 1/2 pound squid, cleaned and sliced into rings
- 1 cup frozen peas
- 1/4 cup chopped fresh parsley
- Lemon wedges for serving

Instructions

1. Heat the olive oil in a large paella pan or deep skillet over medium heat.
2. Add the onion, red bell pepper, and garlic, and sauté until softened, about 5 minutes.
3. Stir in the Arborio rice, smoked paprika, and turmeric, cooking for 2 minutes until the rice is coated.
4. Add the broth and diced tomatoes, bringing to a simmer. Cook, uncovered, for about 20 minutes, stirring occasionally, until the rice is tender and the liquid is mostly absorbed.
5. Add the shrimp, mussels, squid, and peas. Cover and cook for an additional 10 minutes, until the seafood is cooked through and the mussels have opened.
6. Garnish with chopped parsley and serve with lemon wedges.

Nutrition Info (per serving)

- Calories: 380
- Protein: 25g
- Carbohydrates: 45g
- Fat: 10g
- Fiber: 4g
- Sugars: 5g
- Sodium: 360mg

7. Crab Stuffed Avocados

Servings: 4
Cooking Time: 10 minutes
Ingredients

- 2 ripe avocados, halved and pitted
- 1 cup lump crab meat
- 1/4 cup Greek yogurt
- 1 tablespoon lime juice
- 1 teaspoon Dijon mustard
- 1 tablespoon chopped fresh cilantro
- 1/2 teaspoon smoked paprika

Instructions

1. In a bowl, combine the crab meat, Greek yogurt, lime juice, Dijon mustard, chopped cilantro, and smoked paprika. Mix gently.
2. Scoop out a small amount of avocado flesh to create a larger cavity.
3. Fill each avocado half with the crab mixture.
4. Serve immediately.

Nutrition Info (per serving)

- Calories: 240
- Protein: 14g
- Carbohydrates: 10g
- Fat: 18g
- Fiber: 7g
- Sugars: 1g
- Sodium: 360mg

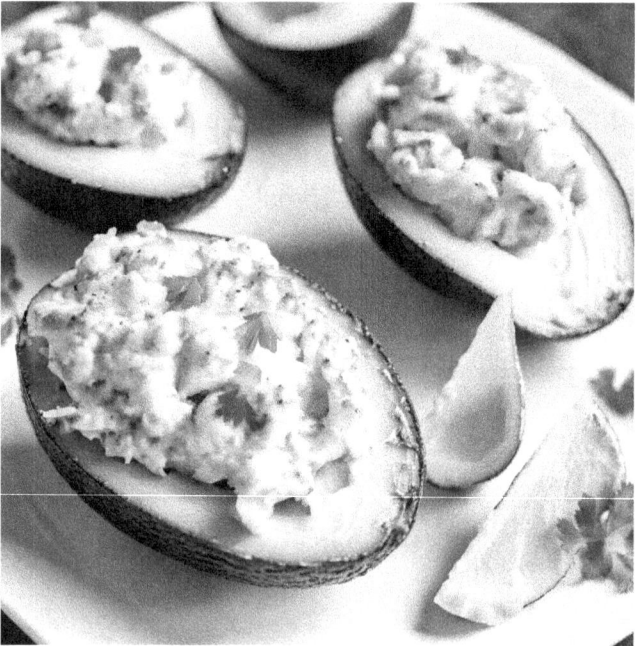

8. Asian Salmon Bowl

Servings: 4
Cooking Time: 25 minutes
Ingredients

- 4 salmon fillets (6 ounces each)
- 1 tablespoon sesame oil
- 2 tablespoons low-sodium soy sauce
- 1 tablespoon honey
- 1 teaspoon grated fresh ginger
- 1 teaspoon sesame seeds
- 1 cup quinoa, cooked
- 1 cup shredded carrots
- 1 cup sliced cucumber
- 1 avocado, sliced
- 1/4 cup chopped green onions

Instructions

1. Preheat the oven to 375°F (190°C).
2. In a small bowl, mix the sesame oil, soy sauce, honey, and grated ginger.
3. Place the salmon fillets on a baking sheet and brush with the soy sauce mixture.
4. Bake for 15-20 minutes, until the salmon is cooked through and flakes easily with a fork.
5. Divide the cooked quinoa between four bowls.
6. Top each bowl with a salmon fillet, shredded carrots, sliced cucumber, and avocado slices.
7. Sprinkle with sesame seeds and chopped green onions.
8. Serve immediately.

Nutrition Info (per serving)

- Calories: 480
- Protein: 32g
- Carbohydrates: 30g
- Fat: 25g
- Fiber: 8g
- Sugars: 8g
- Sodium: 450mg

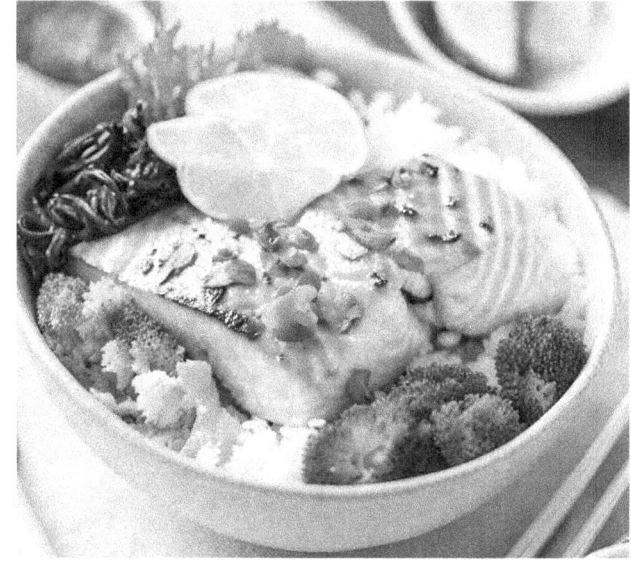

9. Mediterranean Baked Trout

Servings: 4
Cooking Time: 30 minutes
Ingredients

- 4 trout fillets (6 ounces each)
- 2 tablespoons olive oil
- 1 tablespoon lemon juice
- 1 teaspoon dried oregano
- 1 teaspoon garlic powder
- 1 cup cherry tomatoes, halved
- 1/4 cup Kalamata olives, pitted and halved
- 1/4 cup crumbled feta cheese
- Fresh parsley for garnish

Instructions

1. Preheat the oven to 375°F (190°C).
2. In a small bowl, mix the olive oil, lemon juice, dried oregano, and garlic powder.
3. Place the trout fillets in a baking dish and brush with the olive oil mixture.
4. Arrange the cherry tomatoes and Kalamata olives around the trout fillets.
5. Bake for 20 minutes, until the trout is cooked through and flakes easily with a fork.
6. Sprinkle with crumbled feta cheese and garnish with fresh parsley.
7. Serve immediately.

Nutrition Info (per serving)

- Calories: 350
- Protein: 30g
- Carbohydrates: 5g
- Fat: 22g
- Fiber: 2g
- Sugars: 3g
- Sodium: 400mg

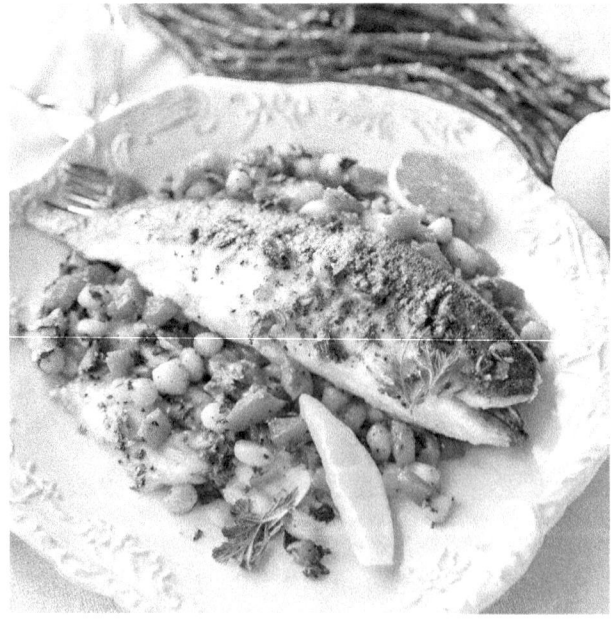

10. Pesto Grilled Shrimp

Servings: 4
Cooking Time: 15 minutes
Ingredients

- 1 pound large shrimp, peeled and deveined
- 1/4 cup pesto sauce
- 1 tablespoon olive oil
- 1 tablespoon lemon juice

Instructions

1. Preheat the grill to medium-high heat.
2. In a bowl, combine the shrimp, pesto sauce, olive oil, and lemon juice. Toss to coat evenly.
3. Thread the shrimp onto skewers.
4. Grill the shrimp for 2-3 minutes on each side, until pink and opaque.
5. Serve immediately.

Nutrition Info (per serving)

- Calories: 220
- Protein: 25g
- Carbohydrates: 2g
- Fat: 12g
- Fiber: 0g
- Sugars: 0g
- Sodium: 350mg

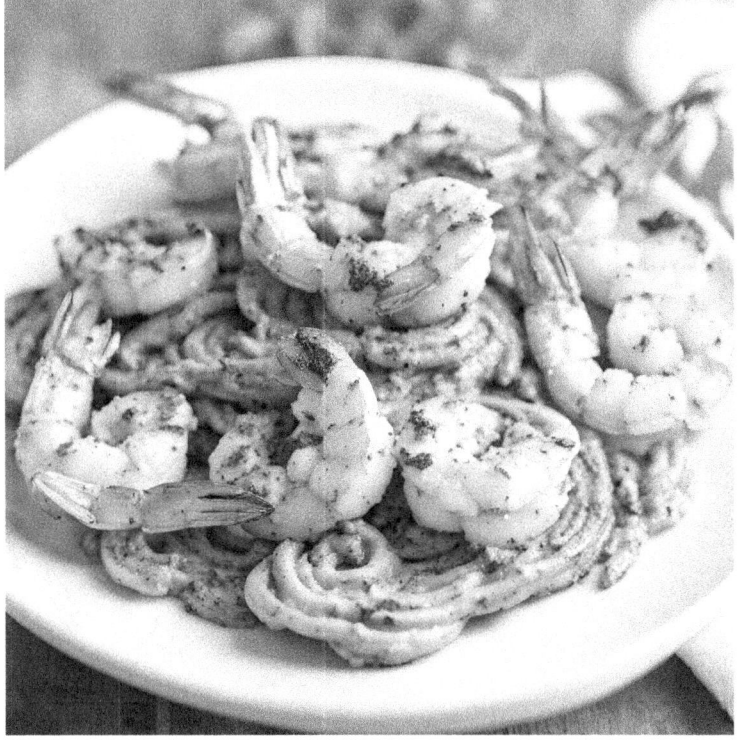

11. Baked Tilapia with Dill Sauce

Servings: 4
Cooking Time: 20 minutes
Ingredients

Tilapia:

- 4 tilapia fillets (6 ounces each)
- 1 tablespoon olive oil
- 1 teaspoon ground paprika
- 1 teaspoon garlic powder

Dill Sauce:

- 1/2 cup Greek yogurt
- 1 tablespoon fresh dill, chopped
- 1 tablespoon lemon juice
- 1 teaspoon Dijon mustard

Instructions

1. Preheat the oven to 375°F (190°C).
2. Place the tilapia fillets in a baking dish and brush with olive oil.
3. Sprinkle with paprika and garlic powder.
4. Bake for 15-20 minutes, until the tilapia is cooked through and flakes easily with a fork.
5. In a small bowl, mix the Greek yogurt, chopped dill, lemon juice, and Dijon mustard.
6. Serve the tilapia fillets with the dill sauce.

Nutrition Info (per serving)

- Calories: 220
- Protein: 32g
- Carbohydrates: 3g
- Fat: 9g
- Fiber: 0g
- Sugars: 2g
- Sodium: 180mg

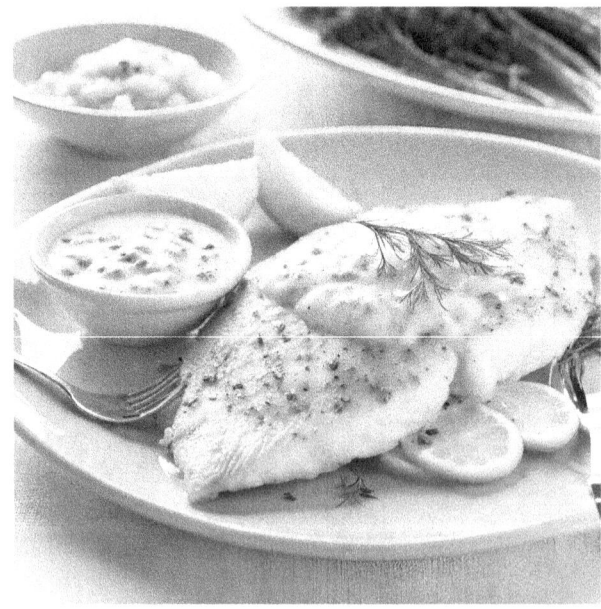

12. Mackerel in Tomato Sauce

Servings: 4

Cooking Time: 25 minutes

Ingredients

- 4 mackerel fillets (6 ounces each)
- 1 tablespoon olive oil
- 1 onion, chopped
- 2 garlic cloves, minced
- 1 can (14.5 ounces) diced tomatoes
- 1 teaspoon dried oregano
- 1 teaspoon paprika
- 1/4 teaspoon red pepper flakes
- 1 tablespoon lemon juice
- Fresh parsley for garnish

Instructions

1. Heat the olive oil in a large skillet over medium heat.
2. Add the chopped onion and garlic, and sauté until softened, about 5 minutes.
3. Add the diced tomatoes, dried oregano, paprika, and red pepper flakes. Bring to a simmer and cook for 10 minutes.
4. Place the mackerel fillets in the skillet, spooning some sauce over them.
5. Cover and cook for 10-12 minutes, until the fish is cooked through and flakes easily with a fork.
6. Drizzle with lemon juice and garnish with fresh parsley.
7. Serve immediately.

Nutrition Info (per serving)

- Calories: 320
- Protein: 28g
- Carbohydrates: 10g
- Fat: 18g
- Fiber: 2g
- Sugars: 5g
- Sodium: 180mg

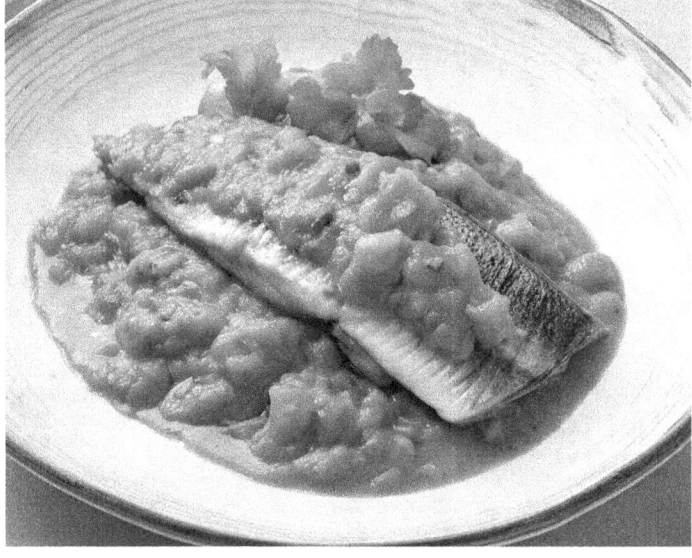

13. Seared Tuna Steaks
Servings: 4
Cooking Time: 10 minutes
Ingredients

- 4 tuna steaks (6 ounces each)
- 1 tablespoon olive oil
- 1 teaspoon sesame oil
- 2 tablespoons low-sodium soy sauce
- 1 tablespoon lime juice
- 1 teaspoon grated fresh ginger
- 1 tablespoon sesame seeds

Instructions

1. In a small bowl, mix the sesame oil, soy sauce, lime juice, and grated ginger.
2. Brush the tuna steaks with the soy sauce mixture.
3. Heat the olive oil in a large skillet over medium-high heat.
4. Sear the tuna steaks for 2-3 minutes on each side, until cooked to desired doneness.
5. Sprinkle with sesame seeds and serve immediately.

Nutrition Info (per serving)

- Calories: 280
- Protein: 36g
- Carbohydrates: 2g
- Fat: 14g
- Fiber: 0g
- Sugars: 0g
- Sodium: 320mg

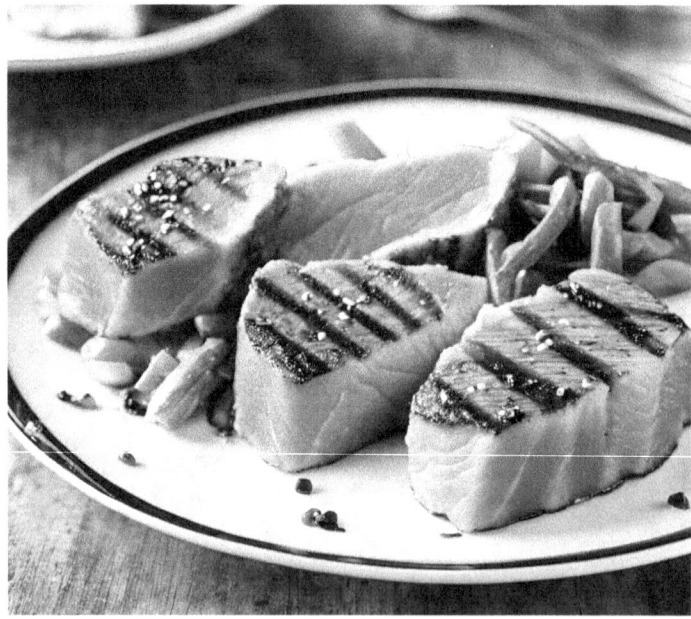

14. Salmon and Spinach Quiche

Servings: 6
Cooking Time: 45 minutes
Ingredients

- 1 whole grain pie crust
- 1 tablespoon olive oil
- 1 small onion, chopped
- 1 cup fresh spinach, chopped
- 1 cup cooked salmon, flaked
- 4 large eggs
- 1 cup unsweetened almond milk
- 1/2 teaspoon dried dill
- 1/4 teaspoon ground nutmeg
- Fresh chives for garnish

Instructions

1. Preheat the oven to 350°F (175°C).
2. Heat the olive oil in a skillet over medium heat. Add the chopped onion and sauté until softened, about 5 minutes.
3. Add the spinach and cook until wilted, about 2 minutes.
4. Spread the cooked spinach and onion mixture evenly over the bottom of the pie crust. Top with flaked salmon.
5. In a bowl, whisk together the eggs, almond milk, dried dill, and ground nutmeg.
6. Pour the egg mixture over the spinach and salmon in the pie crust.
7. Bake for 30-35 minutes, until the quiche is set and golden brown.
8. Garnish with fresh chives and serve warm.

Nutrition Info (per serving)

- Calories: 260
- Protein: 15g
- Carbohydrates: 18g
- Fat: 15g
- Fiber: 3g
- Sugars: 2g
- Sodium: 200mg

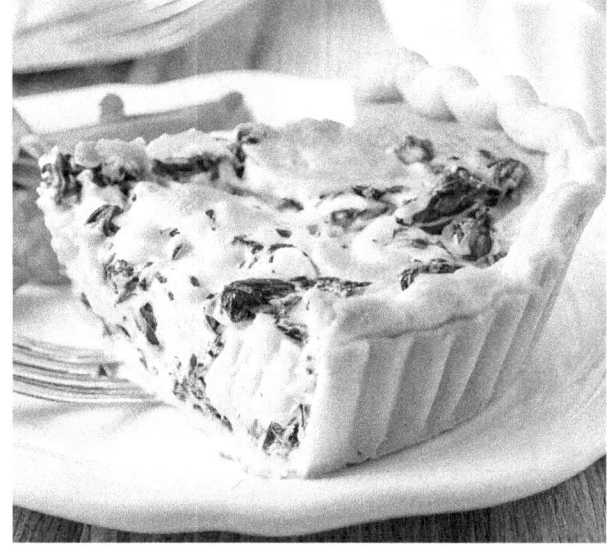

15. Catfish Amandine

Servings: 4

Cooking Time: 20 minutes

Ingredients

- 4 catfish fillets (6 ounces each)
- 2 tablespoons olive oil
- 1/4 cup slivered almonds
- 1 tablespoon lemon juice
- 1 tablespoon chopped fresh parsley

Instructions

1. Heat 1 tablespoon of olive oil in a large skillet over medium heat.
2. Add the catfish fillets and cook for about 4-5 minutes on each side, until the fish is golden brown and cooked through. Remove from the skillet and keep warm.
3. In the same skillet, add the remaining 1 tablespoon of olive oil and slivered almonds. Cook until the almonds are golden brown, about 2 minutes.
4. Drizzle with lemon juice and sprinkle with fresh parsley.
5. Pour the almond mixture over the catfish fillets and serve immediately.

Nutrition Info (per serving)

- Calories: 320
- Protein: 28g
- Carbohydrates: 2g
- Fat: 22g
- Fiber: 1g
- Sugars: 0g
- Sodium: 160mg

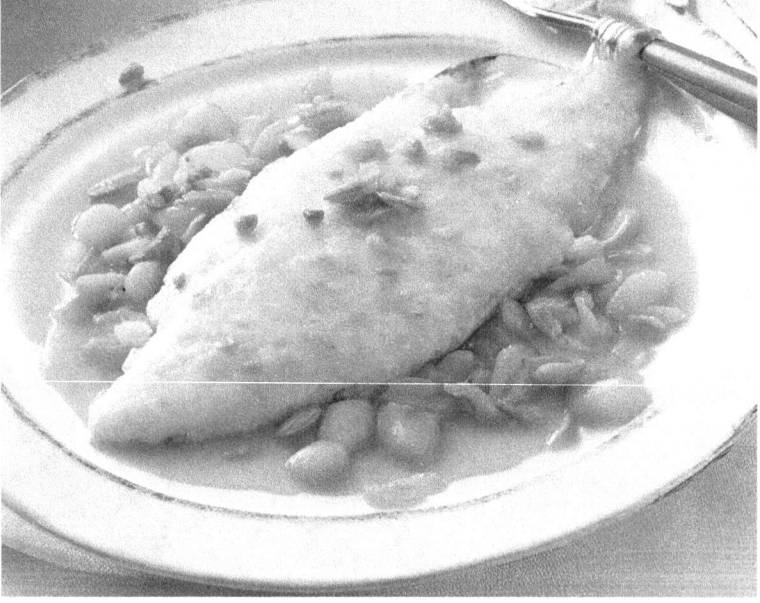

16. Scallop and Asparagus Risotto

Servings: 4
Cooking Time: 35 minutes
Ingredients

- 1 pound large scallops
- 2 tablespoons olive oil, divided
- 1 small onion, chopped
- 1 1/2 cups Arborio rice
- 4 cups low-sodium vegetable broth, warmed
- 1/2 cup white wine (optional)
- 1 cup asparagus, trimmed and cut into 1-inch pieces
- 1/4 cup grated Parmesan cheese
- 1 tablespoon lemon juice
- Fresh parsley for garnish

Instructions

1. Heat 1 tablespoon of olive oil in a large skillet over medium heat. Add the scallops and cook for 2-3 minutes on each side until golden brown and opaque. Remove from the skillet and keep warm.
2. In the same skillet, heat the remaining 1 tablespoon of olive oil. Add the chopped onion and sauté until softened, about 5 minutes.
3. Stir in the Arborio rice and cook for 2 minutes until the rice is lightly toasted.
4. Add the white wine, if using, and cook until absorbed. Gradually add the warm vegetable broth, one cup at a time, stirring constantly until each addition is absorbed before adding the next.
5. After about 15 minutes, stir in the asparagus pieces and continue cooking until the rice is creamy and tender, about 5-10 minutes.
6. Stir in the Parmesan cheese and lemon juice.
7. Serve the risotto topped with the cooked scallops and garnish with fresh parsley.

Nutrition Info (per serving)

- Calories: 400
- Protein: 25g
- Carbohydrates: 48g
- Fat: 12g
- Fiber: 3g
- Sugars: 4g
- Sodium: 300mg

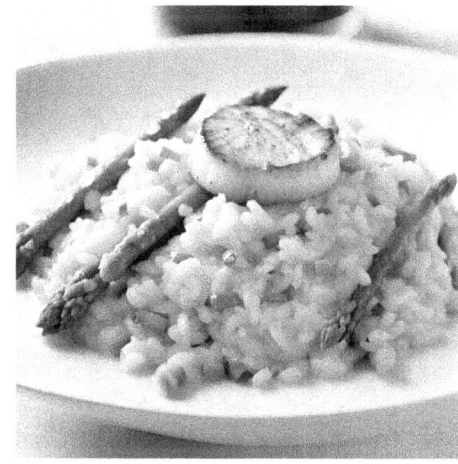

17. Spicy Shrimp and Kale Stir Fry

Servings: 4

Cooking Time: 20 minutes

Ingredients

- 1 pound large shrimp, peeled and deveined
- 2 tablespoons olive oil
- 1 small onion, chopped
- 2 garlic cloves, minced
- 1 red bell pepper, sliced
- 4 cups chopped kale
- 1 tablespoon low-sodium soy sauce
- 1 tablespoon sriracha sauce
- 1 tablespoon honey
- 1 teaspoon grated fresh ginger
- 1/4 cup chopped green onions

Instructions

1. Heat 1 tablespoon of olive oil in a large skillet or wok over medium-high heat. Add the shrimp and cook for 2-3 minutes until pink and opaque. Remove from the skillet and keep warm.
2. In the same skillet, heat the remaining 1 tablespoon of olive oil. Add the chopped onion, garlic, and red bell pepper. Cook for about 5 minutes until the vegetables are tender.
3. Add the chopped kale and cook for an additional 3-4 minutes until wilted.
4. In a small bowl, mix the soy sauce, sriracha sauce, honey, and grated ginger. Pour over the vegetables and stir to combine.
5. Return the cooked shrimp to the skillet and toss to coat with the sauce. Cook for another 1-2 minutes until heated through.
6. Garnish with chopped green onions and serve immediately.

Nutrition Info (per serving)

- Calories: 280
- Protein: 25g
- Carbohydrates: 18g
- Fat: 12g
- Fiber: 4g
- Sugars: 8g
- Sodium: 420mg

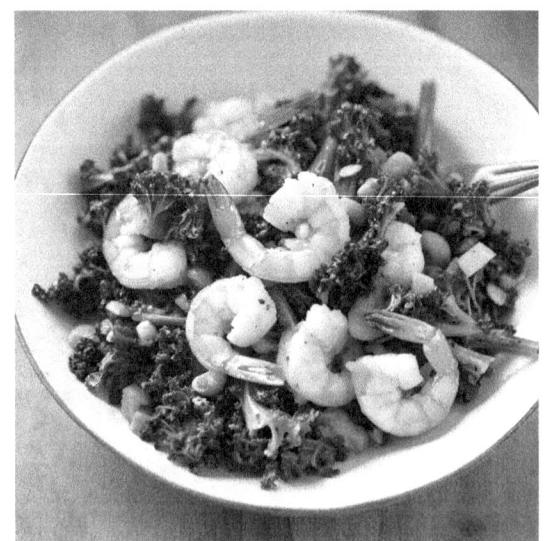

18. Grilled Mackerel with Herb Salad

Servings: 4
Cooking Time: 20 minutes
Ingredients

- 4 mackerel fillets (6 ounces each)
- 2 tablespoons olive oil
- 1 tablespoon lemon juice
- 1 teaspoon dried oregano
- 1 teaspoon ground cumin
- 2 cups mixed herbs (parsley, cilantro, mint), chopped
- 1 cup cherry tomatoes, halved
- 1/2 red onion, thinly sliced
- 1 tablespoon balsamic vinegar

Instructions

1. Preheat the grill to medium-high heat.
2. In a small bowl, mix the olive oil, lemon juice, dried oregano, and ground cumin.
3. Brush the mackerel fillets with the olive oil mixture.
4. Grill the mackerel for 4-5 minutes on each side until cooked through and flaky.
5. In a large bowl, combine the mixed herbs, cherry tomatoes, red onion, and balsamic vinegar. Toss to combine.
6. Serve the grilled mackerel with the herb salad.

Nutrition Info (per serving)

- Calories: 320
- Protein: 28g
- Carbohydrates: 6g
- Fat: 20g
- Fiber: 2g
- Sugars: 3g
- Sodium: 90mg

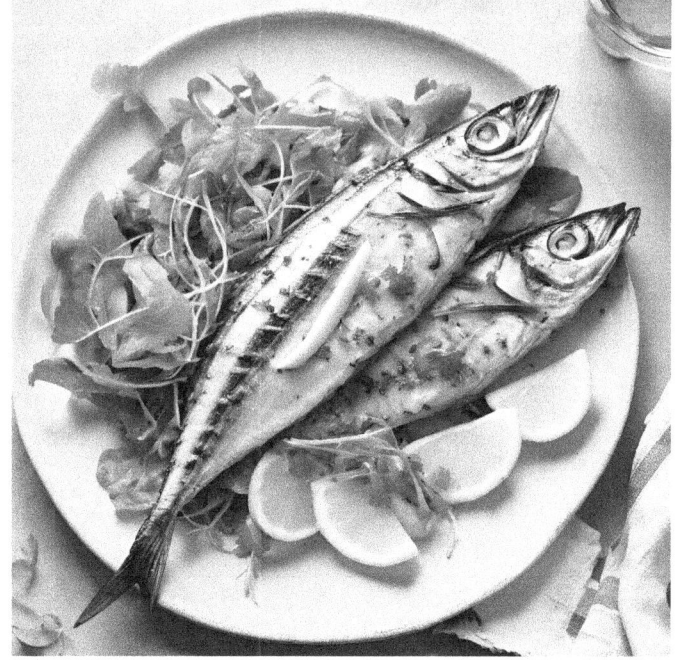

19. Squid Ink Pasta

Servings: 4
Cooking Time: 25 minutes
Ingredients

- 12 ounces squid ink pasta
- 1 pound squid, cleaned and cut into rings
- 2 tablespoons olive oil
- 3 garlic cloves, minced
- 1/4 teaspoon red pepper flakes
- 1/2 cup white wine
- 1 cup cherry tomatoes, halved
- 1/4 cup chopped fresh parsley
- Lemon wedges for serving

Instructions

1. Cook the squid ink pasta according to package instructions. Drain and set aside.
2. Heat the olive oil in a large skillet over medium heat. Add the minced garlic and red pepper flakes, and sauté for 1-2 minutes until fragrant.
3. Add the squid rings and cook for 3-4 minutes until opaque.
4. Pour in the white wine and add the cherry tomatoes. Cook for an additional 5 minutes until the tomatoes are softened.
5. Toss the cooked pasta with the squid and tomato mixture.
6. Garnish with chopped fresh parsley and serve with lemon wedges.

Nutrition Info (per serving)

- Calories: 350
- Protein: 25g
- Carbohydrates: 50g
- Fat: 8g
- Fiber: 3g
- Sugars: 2g
- Sodium: 180mg

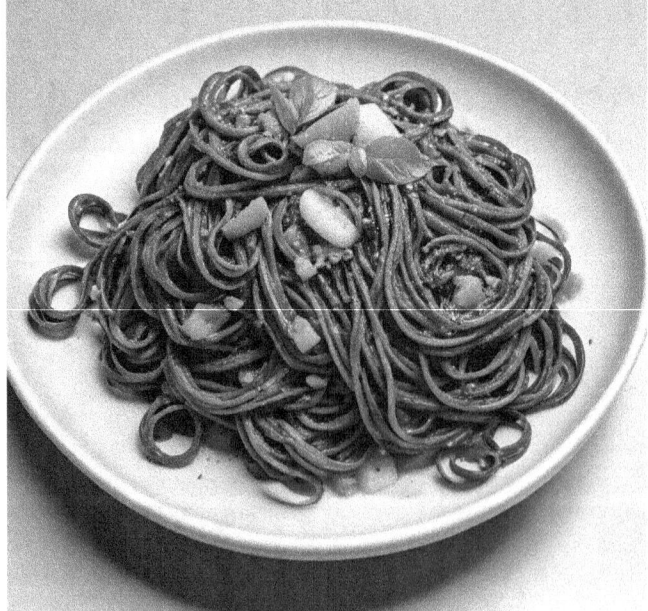

20. Halibut with Tomato Basil Sauce

Servings: 4

Cooking Time: 25 minutes

Ingredients

- 4 halibut fillets (6 ounces each)
- 2 tablespoons olive oil
- 1 onion, chopped
- 3 garlic cloves, minced
- 2 cups cherry tomatoes, halved
- 1/4 cup fresh basil leaves, chopped
- 1 tablespoon lemon juice
- Fresh basil leaves for garnish

Instructions

1. Preheat the oven to 375°F (190°C).
2. Heat 1 tablespoon of olive oil in a large skillet over medium heat. Add the chopped onion and minced garlic, and sauté for 5 minutes until softened.
3. Add the cherry tomatoes and cook for 5 minutes until softened. Stir in the chopped basil and lemon juice.
4. Place the halibut fillets in a baking dish and brush with the remaining 1 tablespoon of olive oil.
5. Pour the tomato basil sauce over the halibut.
6. Bake for 15-20 minutes until the halibut is cooked through and flakes easily with a fork.
7. Garnish with fresh basil leaves and serve immediately.

Nutrition Info (per serving)

- Calories: 310
- Protein: 34g
- Carbohydrates: 8g
- Fat: 16g
- Fiber: 2g
- Sugars: 5g
- Sodium: 120mg

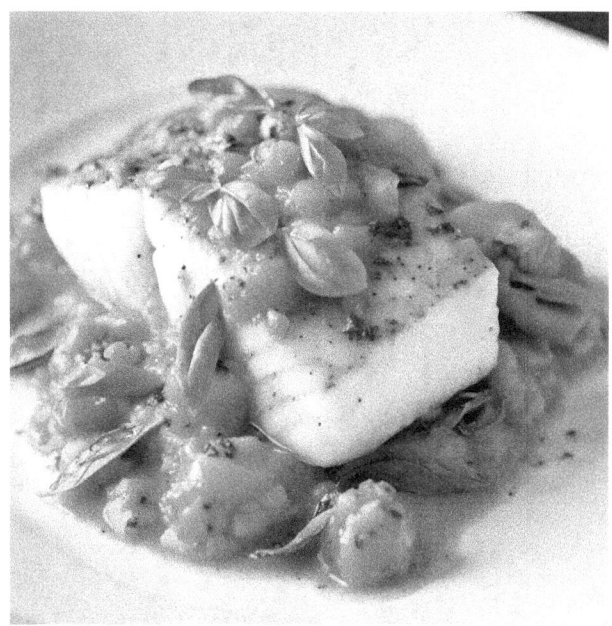

21. Poached Trout with Vegetables

Servings: 4

Cooking Time: 30 minutes

Ingredients

- 4 trout fillets (6 ounces each)
- 4 cups low-sodium vegetable broth
- 1 cup white wine (optional)
- 2 carrots, sliced
- 1 zucchini, sliced
- 1 leek, sliced
- 1 tablespoon lemon juice
- Fresh dill for garnish

Instructions

1. In a large pot, combine the vegetable broth and white wine (if using). Bring to a simmer over medium heat.
2. Add the sliced carrots, zucchini, and leek. Simmer for 10 minutes until the vegetables are tender.
3. Gently place the trout fillets in the pot and poach for 10-12 minutes until the fish is cooked through and flakes easily with a fork.
4. Remove the trout and vegetables from the pot.
5. Drizzle the trout with lemon juice and garnish with fresh dill.
6. Serve immediately.

Nutrition Info (per serving)

- Calories: 220
- Protein: 30g
- Carbohydrates: 8g
- Fat: 7g
- Fiber: 2g
- Sugars: 4g
- Sodium: 220mg

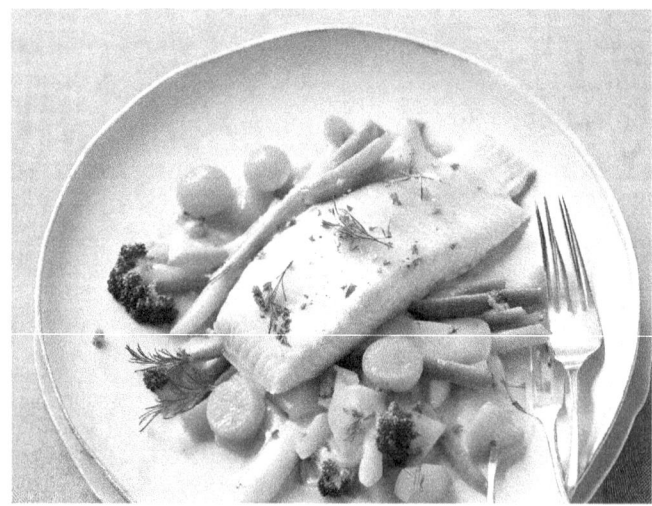

22. Bouillabaisse

Servings: 6

Cooking Time: 45 minutes

Ingredients

- 2 tablespoons olive oil
- 1 onion, chopped
- 2 leeks, sliced
- 3 garlic cloves, minced
- 1 fennel bulb, sliced
- 1 can (14.5 ounces) diced tomatoes
- 4 cups low-sodium fish or vegetable broth
- 1/2 cup white wine (optional)
- 1 teaspoon dried thyme
- 1 teaspoon dried saffron
- 1 bay leaf
- 1 pound white fish fillets, cut into chunks
- 1/2 pound shrimp, peeled and deveined
- 1/2 pound mussels, scrubbed and debearded
- 1/2 pound clams, scrubbed
- Fresh parsley for garnish

Instructions

1. Heat the olive oil in a large pot over medium heat. Add the chopped onion, leeks, garlic, and fennel, and sauté for 10 minutes until softened.
2. Add the diced tomatoes, fish broth, white wine (if using), dried thyme, saffron, and bay leaf. Bring to a simmer and cook for 15 minutes.
3. Add the white fish fillets and cook for 5 minutes.
4. Add the shrimp, mussels, and clams, and cook for an additional 5 minutes until the shellfish open and the shrimp are pink and opaque.
5. Remove the bay leaf and discard.
6. Garnish with fresh parsley and serve immediately.

Nutrition Info (per serving)

- Calories: 320
- Protein: 35g
- Carbohydrates: 12g
- Fat: 10g
- Fiber: 3g
- Sugars: 5g
- Sodium: 360mg

23. Lobster Thermidor

Servings: 4
Cooking Time: 30 minutes

Ingredients

- 2 lobster tails (about 1 pound each)
- 2 tablespoons olive oil
- 1 shallot, minced
- 1/2 cup white wine
- 1/2 cup unsweetened almond milk
- 1 tablespoon Dijon mustard
- 1/4 cup grated Parmesan cheese
- 1 tablespoon fresh parsley, chopped

Instructions

1. Preheat the oven to 375°F (190°C).
2. Boil the lobster tails in a large pot of water for 8-10 minutes until bright red. Remove from the pot and let cool.
3. Remove the lobster meat from the shells and chop into bite-sized pieces. Set aside.
4. Heat the olive oil in a skillet over medium heat. Add the minced shallot and sauté for 2-3 minutes until softened.
5. Add the white wine and cook for 2 minutes until reduced by half.
6. Stir in the almond milk and Dijon mustard. Cook for another 2 minutes.
7. Add the chopped lobster meat to the skillet and toss to coat in the sauce.
8. Divide the lobster mixture between four small baking dishes. Top with grated Parmesan cheese.
9. Bake for 10-12 minutes until the cheese is melted and golden.
10. Garnish with fresh parsley and serve immediately.

Nutrition Info (per serving)

- Calories: 300
- Protein: 28g
- Carbohydrates: 5g
- Fat: 18g
- Fiber: 1g
- Sugars: 2g
- Sodium: 380mg

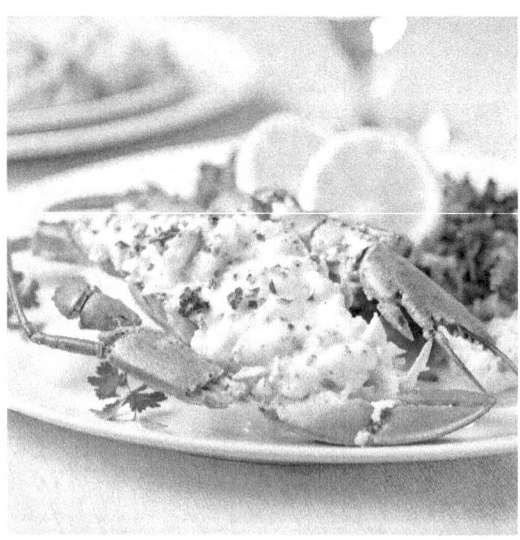

24. Grilled Swordfish with Mango Salsa

Servings: 4

Cooking Time: 20 minutes

Ingredients

- 4 swordfish steaks (6 ounces each)
- 2 tablespoons olive oil
- 1 tablespoon lime juice
- 1 teaspoon ground cumin

Mango Salsa:

- 1 ripe mango, peeled and diced
- 1/2 red bell pepper, diced
- 1/4 cup red onion, finely chopped
- 1/4 cup fresh cilantro, chopped
- 1 tablespoon lime juice

Instructions

1. Preheat the grill to medium-high heat.
2. In a small bowl, mix the olive oil, lime juice, and ground cumin.
3. Brush the swordfish steaks with the olive oil mixture.
4. Grill the swordfish for 4-5 minutes on each side until cooked through and flaky.
5. In a medium bowl, combine the diced mango, red bell pepper, red onion, cilantro, and lime juice. Mix gently.
6. Serve the grilled swordfish topped with mango salsa.

Nutrition Info (per serving)

- Calories: 320
- Protein: 30g
- Carbohydrates: 12g
- Fat: 18g
- Fiber: 2g
- Sugars: 8g
- Sodium: 120mg

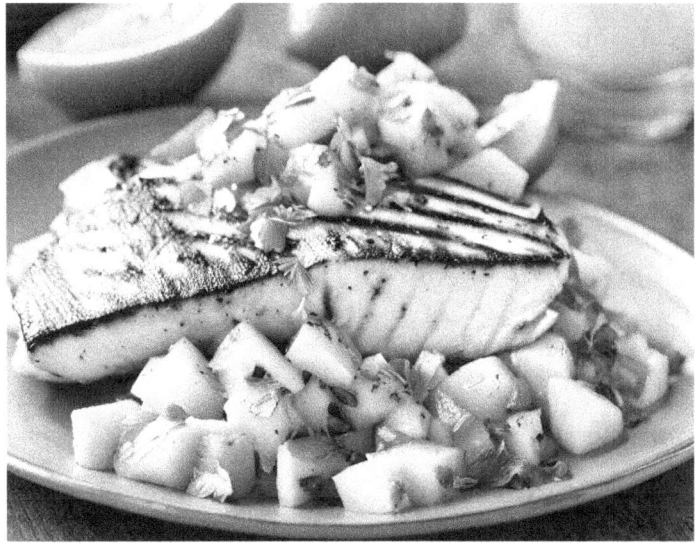

Poultry Recipes

1. Grilled Chicken with Avocado Salsa
Servings: 4
Cooking Time: 25 minutes
Ingredients
Chicken:

- 4 boneless, skinless chicken breasts
- 2 tablespoons olive oil
- 1 tablespoon lemon juice
- 1 teaspoon ground cumin
- 1 teaspoon paprika
- 1/2 teaspoon garlic powder

Avocado Salsa:

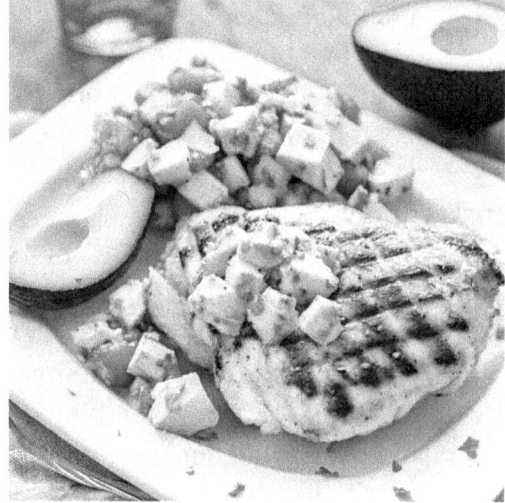

- 2 ripe avocados, diced
- 1 cup cherry tomatoes, quartered
- 1/4 cup red onion, finely chopped
- 1/4 cup fresh cilantro, chopped
- 1 tablespoon lime juice

Instructions

1. Preheat the grill to medium-high heat.
2. In a small bowl, mix the olive oil, lemon juice, ground cumin, paprika, and garlic powder.
3. Brush the chicken breasts with the olive oil mixture.
4. Grill the chicken for 6-7 minutes on each side until cooked through and no longer pink in the center.
5. While the chicken is grilling, prepare the avocado salsa. In a medium bowl, combine the diced avocados, cherry tomatoes, red onion, cilantro, and lime juice. Mix gently.
6. Serve the grilled chicken topped with avocado salsa.

Nutrition Info (per serving)

- Calories: 350
- Protein: 35g
- Carbohydrates: 10g
- Fat: 20g
- Fiber: 7g
- Sugars: 2g
- Sodium: 150mg

2. Baked Turkey Meatballs
Servings: 4
Cooking Time: 30 minutes
Ingredients

- 1 pound ground turkey
- 1/2 cup whole grain breadcrumbs
- 1/4 cup grated Parmesan cheese
- 1/4 cup chopped fresh parsley
- 1 egg, beaten
- 2 garlic cloves, minced
- 1 teaspoon dried oregano
- 1 teaspoon dried basil
- 1/2 teaspoon onion powder

Instructions

1. Preheat the oven to 400°F (200°C).
2. In a large bowl, combine the ground turkey, whole grain breadcrumbs, Parmesan cheese, chopped parsley, beaten egg, minced garlic, dried oregano, dried basil, and onion powder. Mix well.
3. Form the mixture into 16 meatballs and place them on a baking sheet lined with parchment paper.
4. Bake for 20-25 minutes, until the meatballs are cooked through and golden brown.
5. Serve immediately.

Nutrition Info (per serving)

- Calories: 220
- Protein: 25g
- Carbohydrates: 10g
- Fat: 10g
- Fiber: 2g
- Sugars: 1g
- Sodium: 250mg

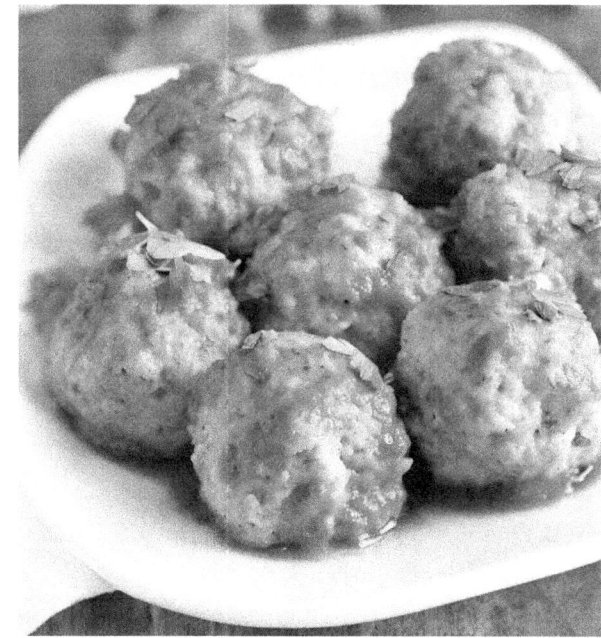

3. Chicken Stir Fry with Broccoli and Ginger

Servings: 4

Cooking Time: 20 minutes

Ingredients

- 1 pound boneless, skinless chicken breasts, sliced into thin strips
- 2 tablespoons olive oil
- 1 tablespoon grated fresh ginger
- 3 garlic cloves, minced
- 1 head broccoli, cut into florets
- 1 red bell pepper, sliced
- 1/4 cup low-sodium soy sauce
- 1 tablespoon honey
- 1 tablespoon sesame seeds

Instructions

1. Heat 1 tablespoon of olive oil in a large skillet or wok over medium-high heat.
2. Add the chicken strips and cook for 5-7 minutes until browned and cooked through. Remove from the skillet and set aside.
3. In the same skillet, heat the remaining 1 tablespoon of olive oil. Add the grated ginger and minced garlic, and sauté for 1-2 minutes until fragrant.
4. Add the broccoli florets and red bell pepper. Stir fry for 5-7 minutes until the vegetables are tender-crisp.
5. In a small bowl, mix the low-sodium soy sauce and honey. Pour the mixture over the vegetables and add the cooked chicken back to the skillet. Toss to combine.
6. Sprinkle with sesame seeds and serve immediately.

Nutrition Info (per serving)

- Calories: 280
- Protein: 30g
- Carbohydrates: 15g
- Fat: 12g
- Fiber: 4g
- Sugars: 7g
- Sodium: 400mg

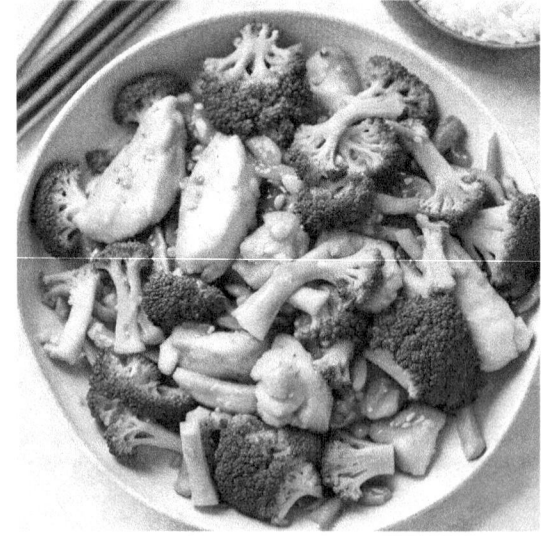

4. Lemon and Rosemary Roast Chicken

Servings: 4

Cooking Time: 1 hour 15 minutes

Ingredients

- 1 whole chicken (about 4 pounds)
- 2 tablespoons olive oil
- 2 lemons, halved
- 4 sprigs fresh rosemary
- 4 garlic cloves, minced
- 1 teaspoon paprika

Instructions

1. Preheat the oven to 375°F (190°C).
2. Rinse the chicken and pat dry with paper towels.
3. Rub the chicken all over with olive oil.
4. Squeeze the juice of one lemon over the chicken, and place the lemon halves inside the cavity along with the rosemary sprigs.
5. Rub the minced garlic and paprika over the chicken.
6. Place the chicken in a roasting pan and roast for about 1 hour 15 minutes, or until the internal temperature reaches 165°F (75°C) and the skin is golden brown.
7. Let the chicken rest for 10 minutes before carving.
8. Serve with lemon wedges.

Nutrition Info (per serving)

- Calories: 400
- Protein: 35g
- Carbohydrates: 3g
- Fat: 28g
- Fiber: 1g
- Sugars: 1g
- Sodium: 180mg

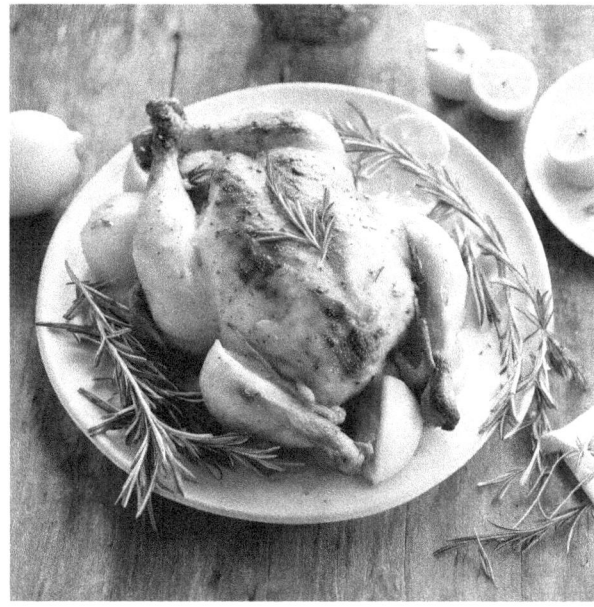

5. Spinach and Feta Stuffed Chicken

Servings: 4

Cooking Time: 40 minutes

Ingredients

- 4 boneless, skinless chicken breasts
- 1 tablespoon olive oil
- 1 cup fresh spinach, chopped
- 1/4 cup crumbled feta cheese
- 2 garlic cloves, minced
- 1 teaspoon dried oregano
- 1 teaspoon paprika

Instructions

1. Preheat the oven to 375°F (190°C).
2. In a small skillet, heat the olive oil over medium heat. Add the chopped spinach and minced garlic, and sauté for 2-3 minutes until the spinach is wilted.
3. Remove from heat and mix in the crumbled feta cheese.
4. Cut a pocket into the side of each chicken breast and stuff with the spinach and feta mixture.
5. Place the stuffed chicken breasts in a baking dish. Sprinkle with dried oregano and paprika.
6. Bake for 30-35 minutes, until the chicken is cooked through and no longer pink in the center.
7. Serve immediately.

Nutrition Info (per serving)

- Calories: 280
- Protein: 35g
- Carbohydrates: 4g
- Fat: 14g
- Fiber: 1g
- Sugars: 1g
- Sodium: 220mg

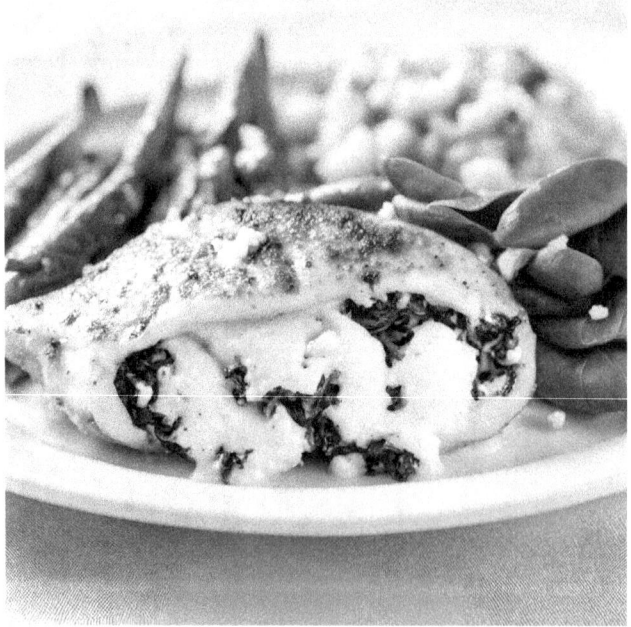

6. Chicken and Quinoa Salad
Servings: 4
Cooking Time: 30 minutes
Ingredients

- 1 cup quinoa
- 2 cups water
- 1 pound boneless, skinless chicken breasts
- 1 tablespoon olive oil
- 1 cup cherry tomatoes, halved
- 1 cucumber, diced
- 1/4 cup red onion, finely chopped
- 1/4 cup crumbled feta cheese
- 2 tablespoons lemon juice
- 2 tablespoons fresh parsley, chopped
- 1 tablespoon fresh mint, chopped

Instructions

1. Rinse the quinoa under cold water. In a medium saucepan, combine the quinoa and water. Bring to a boil, reduce the heat, and simmer for 15 minutes until the water is absorbed and the quinoa is tender. Let cool.
2. While the quinoa is cooking, heat the olive oil in a skillet over medium heat. Add the chicken breasts and cook for 5-7 minutes on each side until browned and cooked through. Let cool, then slice into strips.
3. In a large bowl, combine the cooked quinoa, cherry tomatoes, cucumber, red onion, feta cheese, lemon juice, parsley, and mint. Toss to combine.
4. Add the sliced chicken on top and serve immediately.

Nutrition Info (per serving)

- Calories: 350
- Protein: 30g
- Carbohydrates: 30g
- Fat: 12g
- Fiber: 5g
- Sugars: 3g
- Sodium: 200mg

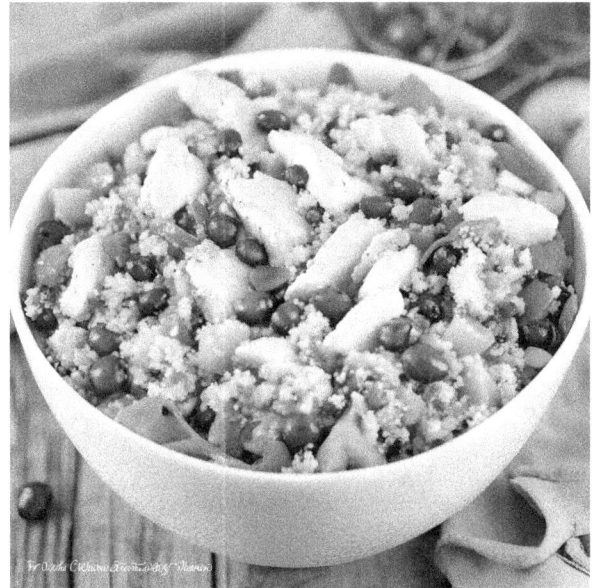

7. Moroccan Chicken Tagine

Servings: 4
Cooking Time: 1 hour
Ingredients

- 1 pound boneless, skinless chicken thighs
- 2 tablespoons olive oil
- 1 onion, chopped
- 3 garlic cloves, minced
- 1 teaspoon ground cumin
- 1 teaspoon ground coriander
- 1 teaspoon ground cinnamon
- 1/2 teaspoon ground ginger
- 1/4 teaspoon turmeric
- 1 cup chicken broth (low sodium)
- 1 can (14.5 ounces) diced tomatoes
- 1 cup carrots, sliced
- 1 cup sweet potatoes, peeled and diced
- 1/4 cup dried apricots, chopped
- 1/4 cup fresh cilantro, chopped

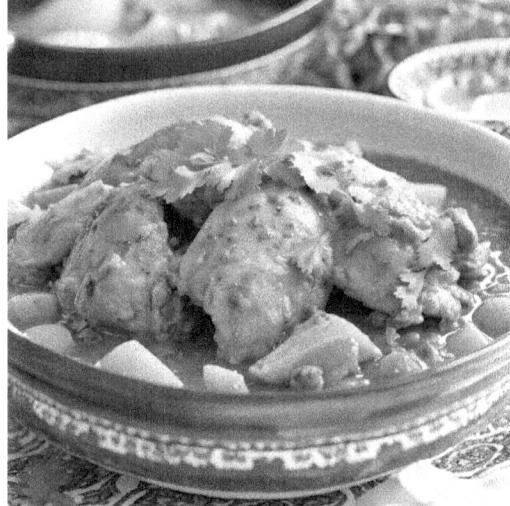

Instructions

1. Heat the olive oil in a large pot or tagine over medium heat. Add the chicken thighs and brown on all sides, about 5-7 minutes. Remove from the pot and set aside.
2. In the same pot, add the onion and garlic, and sauté until softened, about 5 minutes.
3. Stir in the ground cumin, coriander, cinnamon, ginger, and turmeric. Cook for 1 minute until fragrant.
4. Add the chicken broth, diced tomatoes, carrots, sweet potatoes, and dried apricots. Return the chicken to the pot.
5. Bring to a simmer, cover, and cook for 35-40 minutes until the chicken is cooked through and the vegetables are tender.
6. Garnish with fresh cilantro and serve immediately.

Nutrition Info (per serving)

- Calories: 380
- Protein: 28g
- Carbohydrates: 35g
- Fat: 16g
- Fiber: 6g
- Sugars: 14g
- Sodium: 220mg

8. Pesto Chicken Bake

Servings: 4
Cooking Time: 30 minutes
Ingredients

- 4 boneless, skinless chicken breasts
- 1/4 cup basil pesto (store-bought or homemade)
- 1 cup cherry tomatoes, halved
- 1/4 cup grated Parmesan cheese
- 1 tablespoon olive oil

Instructions

1. Preheat the oven to 375°F (190°C).
2. Place the chicken breasts in a baking dish and spread the basil pesto evenly over each piece.
3. Top with halved cherry tomatoes and sprinkle with grated Parmesan cheese.
4. Drizzle with olive oil.
5. Bake for 25-30 minutes, until the chicken is cooked through and the cheese is golden brown.
6. Serve immediately.

Nutrition Info (per serving)

- Calories: 320
- Protein: 35g
- Carbohydrates: 4g
- Fat: 18g
- Fiber: 1g
- Sugars: 2g
- Sodium: 240mg

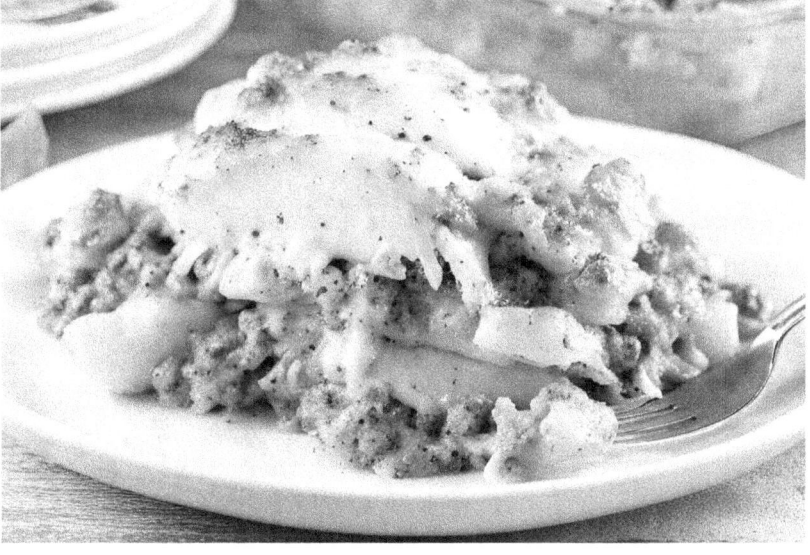

9. Turkey Chili
Servings: 6
Cooking Time: 45 minutes
Ingredients

- 1 pound ground turkey
- 1 tablespoon olive oil
- 1 onion, chopped
- 3 garlic cloves, minced
- 1 bell pepper, chopped
- 1 can (14.5 ounces) diced tomatoes
- 1 can (15 ounces) kidney beans, rinsed and drained
- 1 can (15 ounces) black beans, rinsed and drained
- 2 cups low-sodium chicken broth
- 2 tablespoons chili powder
- 1 teaspoon ground cumin
- 1 teaspoon smoked paprika
- 1/4 teaspoon cayenne pepper (optional)

Instructions

1. Heat the olive oil in a large pot over medium heat. Add the ground turkey and cook until browned, about 5-7 minutes.
2. Add the onion, garlic, and bell pepper, and sauté until softened, about 5 minutes.
3. Stir in the diced tomatoes, kidney beans, black beans, and chicken broth.
4. Add the chili powder, ground cumin, smoked paprika, and cayenne pepper (if using). Stir to combine.
5. Bring to a simmer, cover, and cook for 30 minutes, stirring occasionally.
6. Serve hot.

Nutrition Info (per serving)

- Calories: 280
- Protein: 25g
- Carbohydrates: 30g
- Fat: 8g
- Fiber: 10g
- Sugars: 6g
- Sodium: 300mg

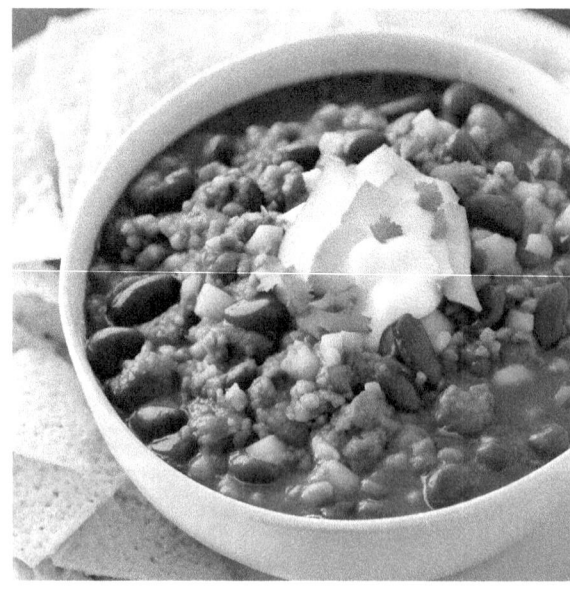

10. Greek Chicken Salad
Servings: 4
Cooking Time: 20 minutes
Ingredients

- 1 pound boneless, skinless chicken breasts, grilled and sliced
- 4 cups mixed greens
- 1 cup cherry tomatoes, halved
- 1 cucumber, diced
- 1/2 cup Kalamata olives, pitted and halved
- 1/4 cup red onion, thinly sliced
- 1/4 cup crumbled feta cheese
- 2 tablespoons olive oil
- 2 tablespoons lemon juice
- 1 teaspoon dried oregano

Instructions

1. In a large bowl, combine the mixed greens, cherry tomatoes, cucumber, Kalamata olives, and red onion.
2. Top with the grilled and sliced chicken.
3. Sprinkle with crumbled feta cheese.
4. In a small bowl, whisk together the olive oil, lemon juice, and dried oregano. Drizzle over the salad.
5. Toss gently to combine and serve immediately.

Nutrition Info (per serving)

- Calories: 350
- Protein: 30g
- Carbohydrates: 10g
- Fat: 20g
- Fiber: 4g
- Sugars: 4g
- Sodium: 280mg

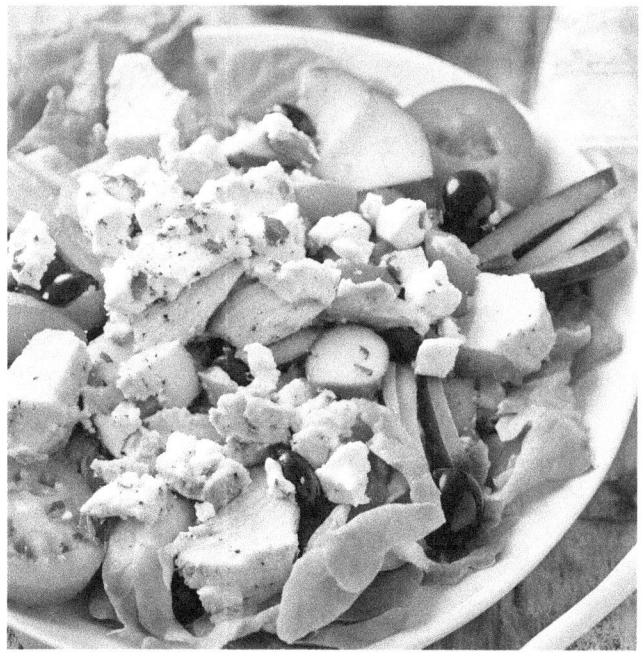

11. Turkey and Spinach Meatloaf

Servings: 4
Cooking Time: 1 hour
Ingredients

- 1 pound ground turkey
- 1 cup fresh spinach, chopped
- 1/2 cup whole grain breadcrumbs
- 1/4 cup grated Parmesan cheese
- 1 egg, beaten
- 2 garlic cloves, minced
- 1 teaspoon dried basil
- 1 teaspoon dried oregano
- 1/2 teaspoon onion powder

Instructions

1. Preheat the oven to 375°F (190°C).
2. In a large bowl, combine the ground turkey, chopped spinach, whole grain breadcrumbs, grated Parmesan cheese, beaten egg, minced garlic, dried basil, dried oregano, and onion powder. Mix well.
3. Form the mixture into a loaf shape and place it in a baking dish.
4. Bake for 50-60 minutes, until the meatloaf is cooked through and golden brown.
5. Let the meatloaf rest for 10 minutes before slicing.
6. Serve immediately.

Nutrition Info (per serving)

- Calories: 280
- Protein: 28g
- Carbohydrates: 12g
- Fat: 14g
- Fiber: 2g
- Sugars: 1g
- Sodium: 240mg

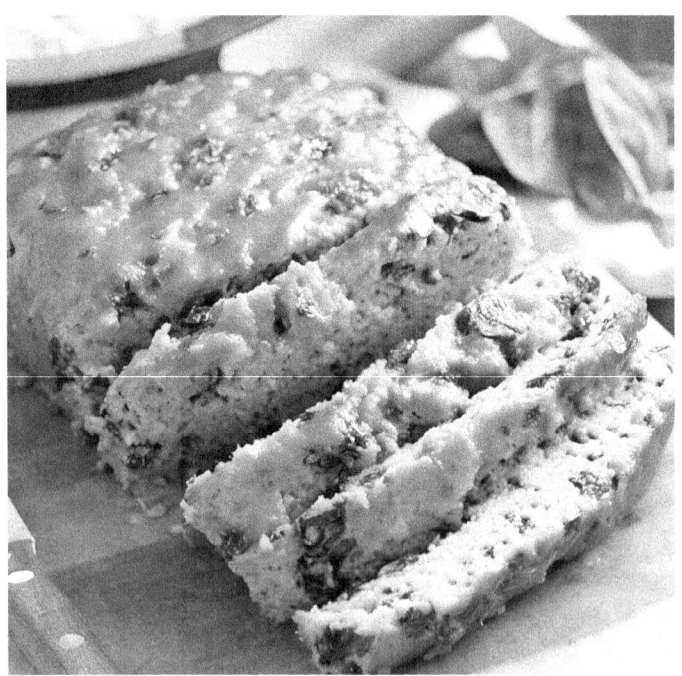

12. Herb-Roasted Turkey Breast

Servings: 4
Cooking Time: 1 hour 30 minutes
Ingredients

- 1 (3-4 pound) turkey breast, bone-in and skin-on
- 2 tablespoons olive oil
- 2 tablespoons fresh rosemary, chopped
- 2 tablespoons fresh thyme, chopped
- 2 tablespoons fresh sage, chopped
- 4 garlic cloves, minced
- 1 tablespoon lemon juice

Instructions

1. Preheat the oven to 375°F (190°C).
2. In a small bowl, combine the olive oil, rosemary, thyme, sage, minced garlic, and lemon juice.
3. Rub the herb mixture all over the turkey breast, making sure to get some under the skin.
4. Place the turkey breast on a rack in a roasting pan.
5. Roast for about 1 hour 30 minutes, or until the internal temperature reaches 165°F (75°C) and the skin is golden brown.
6. Let the turkey rest for 10 minutes before slicing.
7. Serve immediately.

Nutrition Info (per serving)

- Calories: 350
- Protein: 40g
- Carbohydrates: 2g
- Fat: 20g
- Fiber: 0g
- Sugars: 0g
- Sodium: 90mg

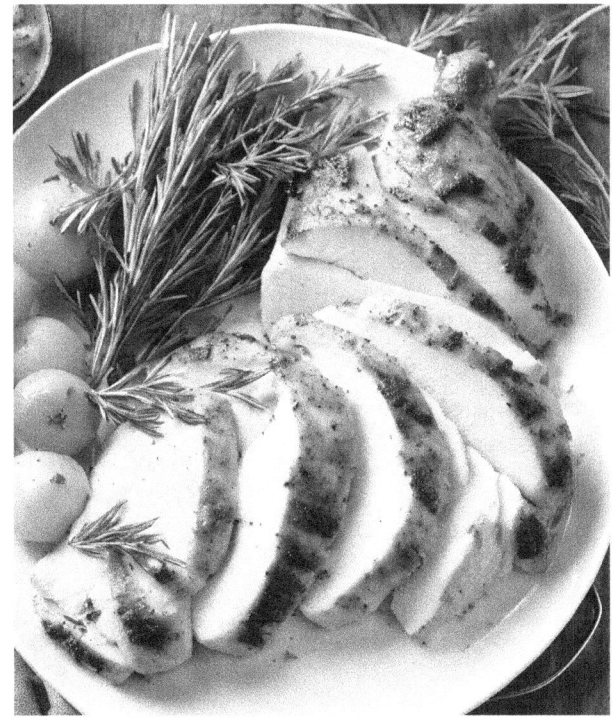

13. Chicken and Sweet Potato Stew

Servings: 4
Cooking Time: 45 minutes
Ingredients

- 1 pound boneless, skinless chicken thighs, cut into bite-sized pieces
- 2 tablespoons olive oil
- 1 onion, chopped
- 3 garlic cloves, minced
- 2 large sweet potatoes, peeled and diced
- 1 can (14.5 ounces) diced tomatoes
- 4 cups low-sodium chicken broth
- 1 teaspoon ground cumin
- 1 teaspoon paprika
- 1/2 teaspoon ground cinnamon
- 1/4 teaspoon cayenne pepper (optional)
- 1/4 cup fresh cilantro, chopped

Instructions

1. Heat the olive oil in a large pot over medium heat. Add the chicken and cook until browned, about 5-7 minutes.
2. Add the onion and garlic, and sauté until softened, about 5 minutes.
3. Stir in the sweet potatoes, diced tomatoes, chicken broth, ground cumin, paprika, ground cinnamon, and cayenne pepper (if using).
4. Bring to a simmer and cook for 30 minutes, until the sweet potatoes are tender and the chicken is cooked through.
5. Garnish with fresh cilantro and serve immediately.

Nutrition Info (per serving)

- Calories: 320
- Protein: 28g
- Carbohydrates: 30g
- Fat: 12g
- Fiber: 5g
- Sugars: 8g
- Sodium: 300mg

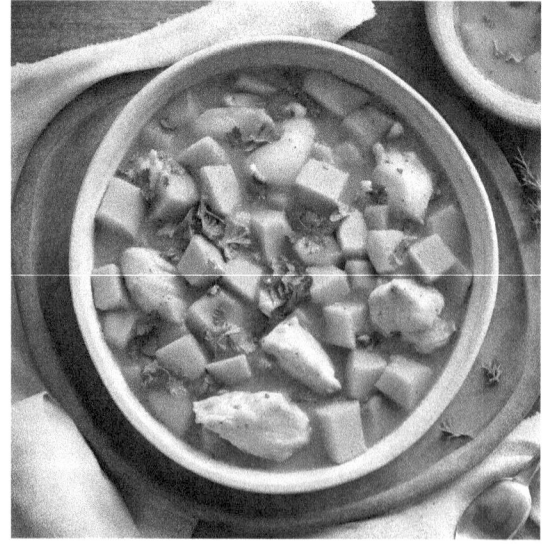

14. Mediterranean Chicken and Grain Bowl

Servings: 4

Cooking Time: 30 minutes

Ingredients

- 1 pound boneless, skinless chicken breasts, grilled and sliced
- 1 cup quinoa, cooked
- 1 cup cherry tomatoes, halved
- 1 cucumber, diced
- 1/4 cup Kalamata olives, pitted and halved
- 1/4 cup red onion, finely chopped
- 1/4 cup crumbled feta cheese
- 2 tablespoons olive oil
- 2 tablespoons lemon juice
- 1 teaspoon dried oregano

Instructions

1. Cook the quinoa according to package instructions. Let cool.
2. In a large bowl, combine the cooked quinoa, cherry tomatoes, cucumber, Kalamata olives, and red onion.
3. Top with the grilled and sliced chicken.
4. Sprinkle with crumbled feta cheese.
5. In a small bowl, whisk together the olive oil, lemon juice, and dried oregano. Drizzle over the bowl.
6. Toss gently to combine and serve immediately.

Nutrition Info (per serving)

- Calories: 380
- Protein: 35g
- Carbohydrates: 30g
- Fat: 14g
- Fiber: 6g
- Sugars: 4g
- Sodium: 300mg

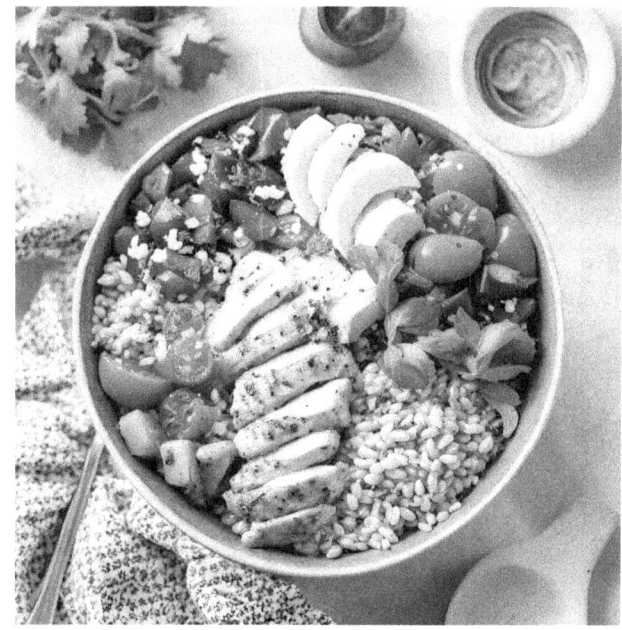

15. Turkey Bolognese

Servings: 4
Cooking Time: 45 minutes
Ingredients

- 1 pound ground turkey
- 2 tablespoons olive oil
- 1 onion, chopped
- 3 garlic cloves, minced
- 1 carrot, diced
- 1 celery stalk, diced
- 1 can (14.5 ounces) diced tomatoes
- 1/4 cup tomato paste
- 1/2 cup low-sodium chicken broth
- 1 teaspoon dried oregano
- 1 teaspoon dried basil
- 1/2 teaspoon ground black pepper
- 1/4 cup fresh parsley, chopped

Instructions

1. Heat the olive oil in a large skillet over medium heat. Add the ground turkey and cook until browned, about 5-7 minutes.
2. Add the onion, garlic, carrot, and celery, and sauté until softened, about 5 minutes.
3. Stir in the diced tomatoes, tomato paste, chicken broth, dried oregano, dried basil, and ground black pepper.
4. Bring to a simmer and cook for 25-30 minutes, until the sauce is thickened.
5. Garnish with fresh parsley and serve over your choice of whole grain pasta or zucchini noodles.

Nutrition Info (per serving)

- Calories: 300
- Protein: 28g
- Carbohydrates: 20g
- Fat: 14g
- Fiber: 4g
- Sugars: 10g
- Sodium: 320mg

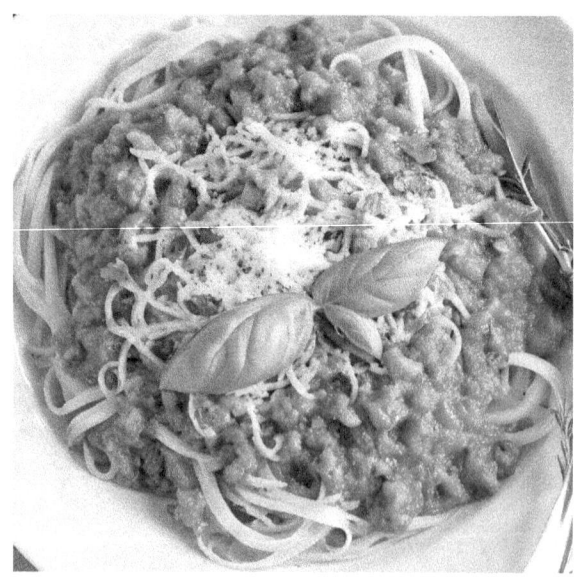

16. Spiced Chicken with Couscous

Servings: 4
Cooking Time: 30 minutes
Ingredients

- 1 pound boneless, skinless chicken thighs, cut into bite-sized pieces
- 2 tablespoons olive oil
- 1 teaspoon ground cumin
- 1 teaspoon ground coriander
- 1/2 teaspoon paprika
- 1/2 teaspoon ground cinnamon
- 1/4 teaspoon ground turmeric
- 1 cup whole wheat couscous
- 1 1/2 cups low-sodium chicken broth
- 1/4 cup chopped fresh parsley
- 1/4 cup chopped fresh mint
- 1/4 cup slivered almonds, toasted
- 1/4 cup raisins

Instructions

1. In a small bowl, combine the ground cumin, ground coriander, paprika, ground cinnamon, and ground turmeric.
2. Toss the chicken pieces with the spice mixture until evenly coated.
3. Heat the olive oil in a large skillet over medium heat. Add the spiced chicken and cook until browned and cooked through, about 10-12 minutes.
4. Meanwhile, bring the chicken broth to a boil in a medium saucepan. Stir in the couscous, cover, and remove from heat. Let stand for 5 minutes, then fluff with a fork.
5. Stir in the chopped parsley, chopped mint, toasted almonds, and raisins.
6. Serve the spiced chicken over the couscous.

Nutrition Info (per serving)

- Calories: 380
- Protein: 28g
- Carbohydrates: 35g
- Fat: 14g
- Fiber: 5g
- Sugars: 8g
- Sodium: 260mg

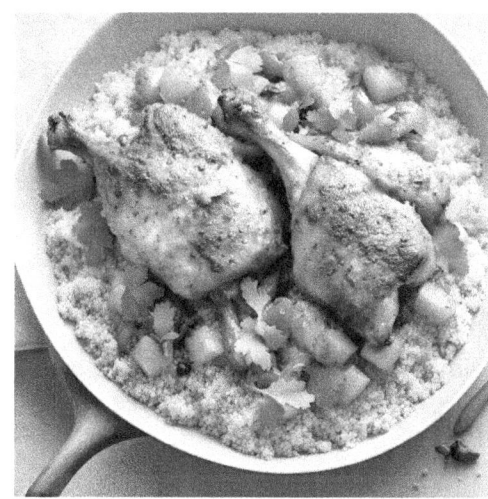

17. Barbecue Chicken Pizza

Servings: 4

Cooking Time: 25 minutes

Ingredients

- 1 whole grain pizza crust
- 1/2 cup barbecue sauce (low sugar)
- 1 cup cooked chicken breast, shredded
- 1/2 red onion, thinly sliced
- 1/2 cup shredded mozzarella cheese
- 1/4 cup chopped fresh cilantro

Instructions

1. Preheat the oven to 425°F (220°C).
2. Spread the barbecue sauce evenly over the pizza crust.
3. Top with shredded chicken, red onion, and shredded mozzarella cheese.
4. Bake in the preheated oven for 12-15 minutes, until the crust is golden and the cheese is bubbly.
5. Remove from the oven and sprinkle with chopped cilantro.
6. Serve immediately.

Nutrition Info (per serving)

- Calories: 320
- Protein: 28g
- Carbohydrates: 35g
- Fat: 10g
- Fiber: 4g
- Sugars: 8g
- Sodium: 400mg

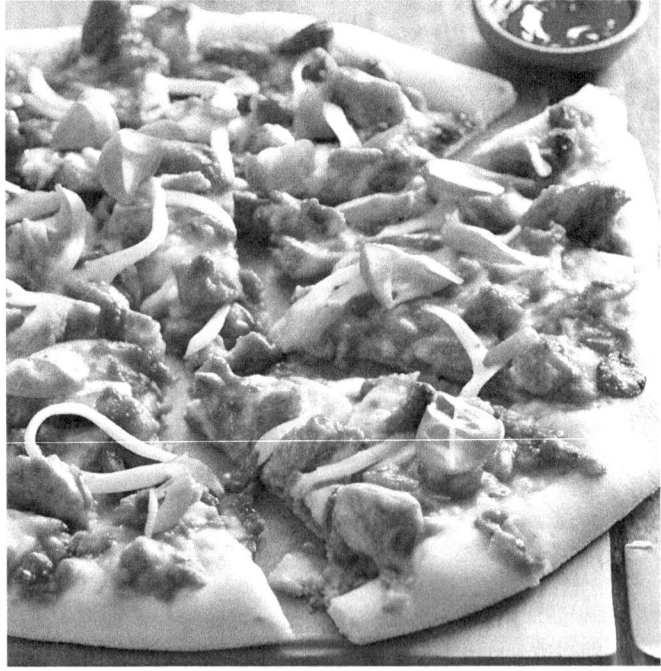

18. Buffalo Chicken Salad

Servings: 4

Cooking Time: 20 minutes

Ingredients

- 1 pound boneless, skinless chicken breasts
- 2 tablespoons olive oil
- 1/4 cup hot sauce (low sodium)
- 4 cups mixed greens
- 1 cup cherry tomatoes, halved
- 1/2 cup celery, sliced
- 1/4 cup crumbled blue cheese
- 2 tablespoons Greek yogurt
- 1 tablespoon lemon juice

Instructions

1. Heat the olive oil in a large skillet over medium heat. Add the chicken breasts and cook for 5-7 minutes on each side until cooked through. Remove from the skillet and let cool, then slice into strips.
2. Toss the sliced chicken with the hot sauce.
3. In a large bowl, combine the mixed greens, cherry tomatoes, and celery.
4. Top with the buffalo chicken and sprinkle with crumbled blue cheese.
5. In a small bowl, mix the Greek yogurt and lemon juice. Drizzle over the salad.
6. Serve immediately.

Nutrition Info (per serving)

- Calories: 280
- Protein: 28g
- Carbohydrates: 8g
- Fat: 16g
- Fiber: 3g
- Sugars: 4g
- Sodium: 450mg

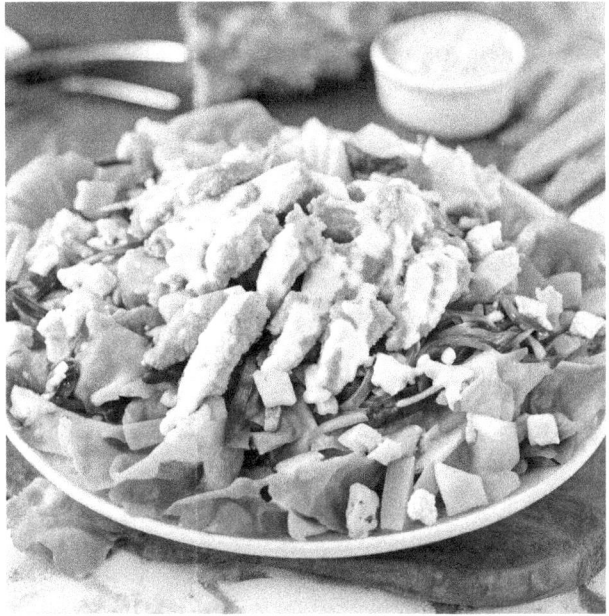

19. Thai Chicken Curry

Servings: 4

Cooking Time: 35 minutes

Ingredients

- 1 pound boneless, skinless chicken thighs, cut into bite-sized pieces
- 2 tablespoons olive oil
- 1 onion, chopped
- 3 garlic cloves, minced
- 1 tablespoon grated fresh ginger
- 1 red bell pepper, sliced
- 1 cup coconut milk (light)
- 1 tablespoon red curry paste
- 1 tablespoon fish sauce
- 1 tablespoon lime juice
- 1/4 cup fresh basil leaves, chopped

Instructions

1. Heat the olive oil in a large pot over medium heat. Add the chicken thighs and cook until browned, about 5-7 minutes. Remove from the pot and set aside.
2. In the same pot, add the onion, garlic, and ginger, and sauté until softened, about 5 minutes.
3. Add the red bell pepper and cook for another 2 minutes.
4. Stir in the coconut milk, red curry paste, fish sauce, and lime juice. Bring to a simmer.
5. Return the chicken to the pot and cook for another 10 minutes, until the chicken is cooked through.
6. Garnish with fresh basil leaves and serve immediately.

Nutrition Info (per serving)

- Calories: 350
- Protein: 28g
- Carbohydrates: 10g
- Fat: 22g
- Fiber: 3g
- Sugars: 4g
- Sodium: 450mg

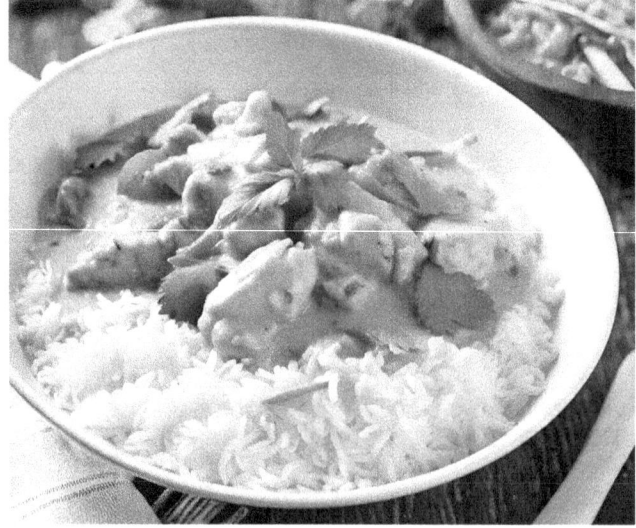

20. Chicken Paprikash
Servings: 4
Cooking Time: 45 minutes
Ingredients

- 1 pound boneless, skinless chicken thighs
- 2 tablespoons olive oil
- 1 onion, chopped
- 3 garlic cloves, minced
- 2 tablespoons sweet paprika
- 1 cup low-sodium chicken broth
- 1 cup diced tomatoes
- 1/2 cup Greek yogurt
- 1 tablespoon chopped fresh parsley

Instructions

1. Heat the olive oil in a large skillet over medium heat. Add the chicken thighs and cook until browned, about 5-7 minutes. Remove from the skillet and set aside.
2. In the same skillet, add the onion and garlic, and sauté until softened, about 5 minutes.
3. Stir in the sweet paprika and cook for 1 minute.
4. Add the chicken broth and diced tomatoes, and bring to a simmer.
5. Return the chicken to the skillet and cook for 25-30 minutes, until the chicken is cooked through and tender.
6. Stir in the Greek yogurt and cook for another 2 minutes.
7. Garnish with fresh parsley and serve immediately.

Nutrition Info (per serving)

- Calories: 320
- Protein: 28g
- Carbohydrates: 12g
- Fat: 18g
- Fiber: 4g
- Sugars: 6g
- Sodium: 350mg

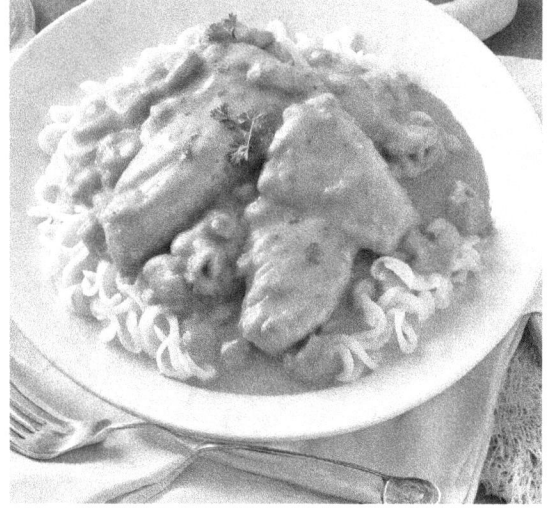

21. Lemon Garlic Chicken Thighs

Servings: 4

Cooking Time: 30 minutes

Ingredients

- 1 pound boneless, skinless chicken thighs
- 2 tablespoons olive oil
- 4 garlic cloves, minced
- 1 tablespoon lemon juice
- 1 tablespoon lemon zest
- 1 teaspoon dried oregano
- Fresh parsley for garnish

Instructions

1. Heat the olive oil in a large skillet over medium heat. Add the chicken thighs and cook until browned, about 5-7 minutes.
2. Add the minced garlic and cook for another 1-2 minutes, until fragrant.
3. Stir in the lemon juice, lemon zest, and dried oregano.
4. Cook for another 15 minutes, until the chicken is cooked through and tender.
5. Garnish with fresh parsley and serve immediately.

Nutrition Info (per serving)

- Calories: 280
- Protein: 28g
- Carbohydrates: 2g
- Fat: 18g
- Fiber: 1g
- Sugars: 0g
- Sodium: 150mg

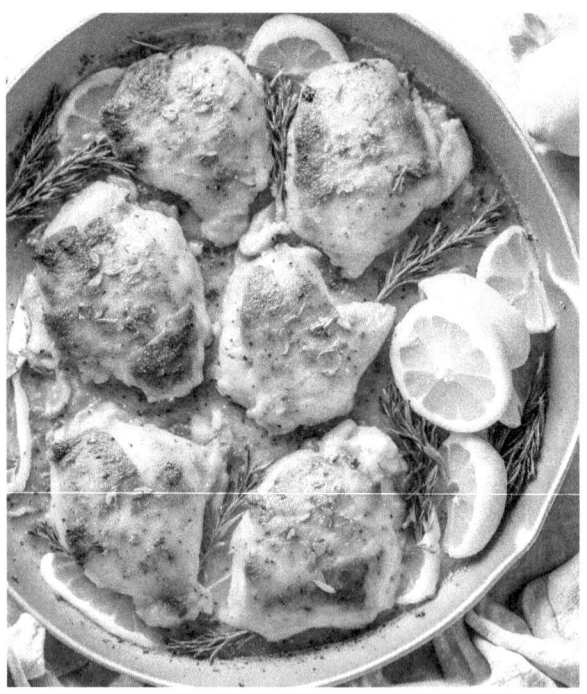

22. Sesame Chicken Salad

Servings: 4
Cooking Time: 25 minutes
Ingredients

- 1 pound boneless, skinless chicken breasts
- 2 tablespoons olive oil
- 2 tablespoons sesame seeds
- 4 cups mixed greens
- 1 cup shredded carrots
- 1 red bell pepper, sliced
- 1/4 cup green onions, chopped
- 2 tablespoons low-sodium soy sauce
- 1 tablespoon rice vinegar
- 1 tablespoon honey
- 1 teaspoon grated fresh ginger

Instructions

1. Heat the olive oil in a skillet over medium heat. Add the chicken breasts and cook for 5-7 minutes on each side until cooked through. Remove from the skillet and let cool, then slice into strips.
2. In the same skillet, toast the sesame seeds for 2-3 minutes until golden brown.
3. In a large bowl, combine the mixed greens, shredded carrots, red bell pepper, and green onions.
4. Top with the sliced chicken and toasted sesame seeds.
5. In a small bowl, whisk together the soy sauce, rice vinegar, honey, and grated ginger. Drizzle over the salad.
6. Toss gently to combine and serve immediately.

Nutrition Info (per serving)

- Calories: 300
- Protein: 28g
- Carbohydrates: 12g
- Fat: 16g
- Fiber: 4g
- Sugars: 6g
- Sodium: 350mg

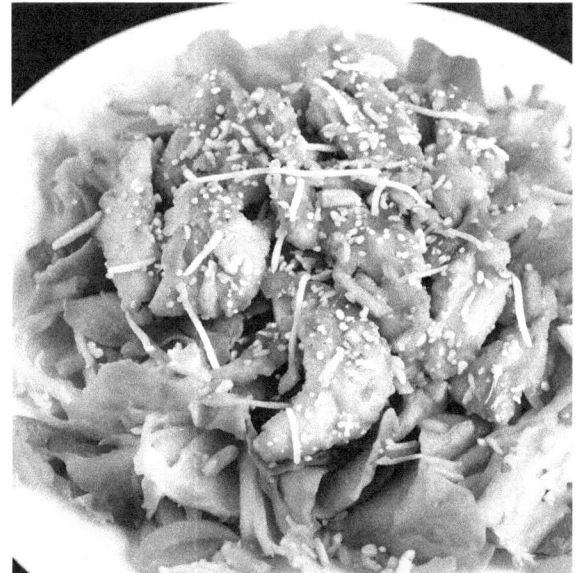

23. Chicken Gyros with Tzatziki
Servings: 4
Cooking Time: 30 minutes
Ingredients
Chicken:

- 1 pound boneless, skinless chicken breasts, sliced
- 2 tablespoons olive oil
- 1 tablespoon lemon juice
- 1 teaspoon dried oregano
- 1 teaspoon ground cumin

Tzatziki:

- 1 cup Greek yogurt
- 1/2 cucumber, grated and drained
- 1 garlic clove, minced
- 1 tablespoon lemon juice
- 1 tablespoon fresh dill, chopped

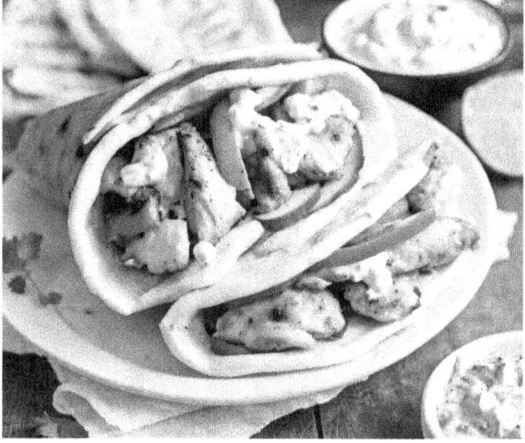

Assembly:

- 4 whole grain pita breads
- 1 cup cherry tomatoes, halved
- 1/2 red onion, thinly sliced
- 1/4 cup crumbled feta cheese

Instructions

1. In a bowl, mix the olive oil, lemon juice, dried oregano, and ground cumin. Toss the chicken slices in the marinade and let sit for 10 minutes.
2. Heat a skillet over medium heat and cook the chicken for 5-7 minutes until cooked through.
3. For the tzatziki, combine the Greek yogurt, grated cucumber, minced garlic, lemon juice, and fresh dill in a bowl. Mix well.
4. To assemble the gyros, place the cooked chicken on the pita breads. Top with cherry tomatoes, red onion, crumbled feta cheese, and a dollop of tzatziki sauce.
5. Serve immediately.

Nutrition Info (per serving)

- Calories: 380
- Protein: 30g
- Carbohydrates: 30g
- Fat: 14g
- Fiber: 6g
- Sugars: 4g
- Sodium: 350mg

24. Balsamic Glazed Chicken

Servings: 4
Cooking Time: 25 minutes
Ingredients

- 1 pound boneless, skinless chicken breasts
- 2 tablespoons olive oil
- 1/4 cup balsamic vinegar
- 2 tablespoons honey
- 1 teaspoon dried thyme
- 1 garlic clove, minced
- Fresh basil for garnish

Instructions

1. Heat the olive oil in a skillet over medium heat. Add the chicken breasts and cook for 5-7 minutes on each side until browned and cooked through. Remove from the skillet and set aside.
2. In the same skillet, add the balsamic vinegar, honey, dried thyme, and minced garlic. Bring to a simmer and cook for 2-3 minutes until thickened.
3. Return the chicken to the skillet and coat with the balsamic glaze.
4. Garnish with fresh basil and serve immediately.

Nutrition Info (per serving)

- Calories: 300
- Protein: 28g
- Carbohydrates: 12g
- Fat: 14g
- Fiber: 1g
- Sugars: 10g
- Sodium: 200mg

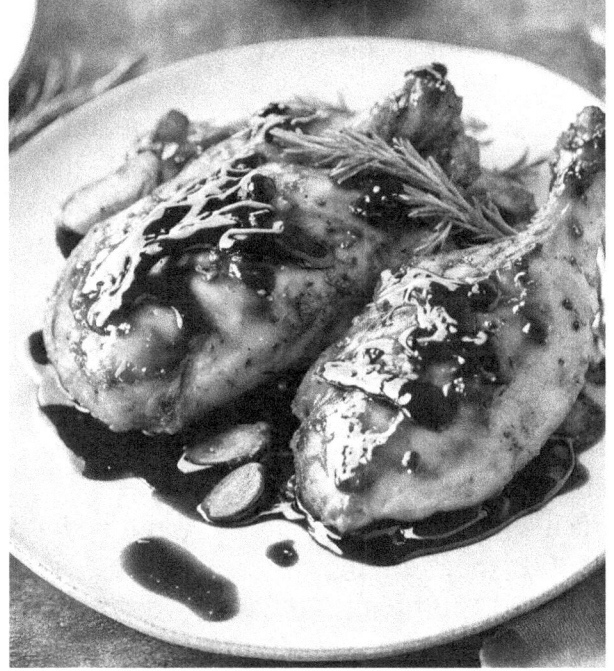

Soup & Stew Recipes

1. Chicken and Kale Stew
Servings: 4
Cooking Time: 45 minutes
Ingredients

- 1 pound boneless, skinless chicken thighs, cut into bite-sized pieces
- 2 tablespoons olive oil
- 1 onion, chopped
- 3 garlic cloves, minced
- 2 carrots, sliced
- 2 celery stalks, sliced
- 1 cup diced tomatoes (canned or fresh)
- 4 cups low-sodium chicken broth
- 4 cups chopped kale, stems removed
- 1 teaspoon dried thyme
- 1 teaspoon dried oregano
- 1 tablespoon lemon juice
- Fresh parsley for garnish

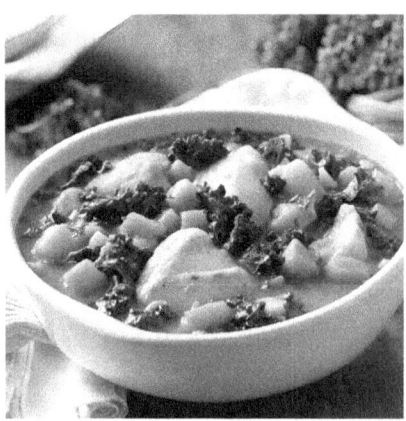

Instructions

1. Heat the olive oil in a large pot over medium heat. Add the chicken thighs and cook until browned, about 5-7 minutes. Remove from the pot and set aside.
2. In the same pot, add the onion, garlic, carrots, and celery. Sauté until softened, about 5 minutes.
3. Stir in the diced tomatoes, chicken broth, dried thyme, and dried oregano. Bring to a simmer.
4. Return the chicken to the pot and cook for 20 minutes.
5. Add the chopped kale and cook for an additional 10 minutes until the kale is tender.
6. Stir in the lemon juice.
7. Garnish with fresh parsley and serve immediately.

Nutrition Info (per serving)

- Calories: 300   Protein: 28g Carbohydrates: 20g   Fat: 12g
- Fiber: 5g
- Sugars: 7g
- Sodium: 300mg

2. Lentil Tomato Soup

Servings: 4
Cooking Time: 40 minutes
Ingredients

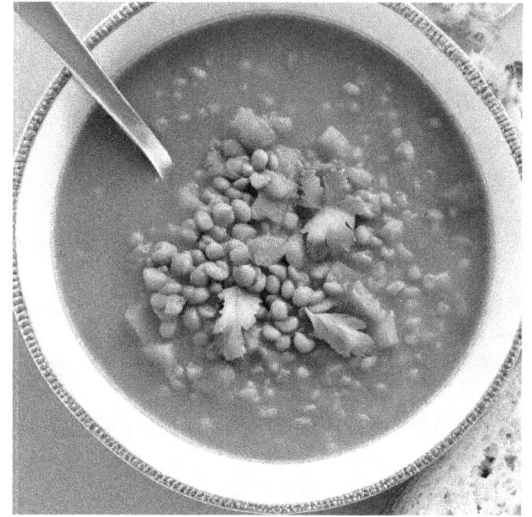

- 1 cup dried lentils, rinsed
- 2 tablespoons olive oil
- 1 onion, chopped
- 3 garlic cloves, minced
- 2 carrots, diced
- 2 celery stalks, diced
- 1 can (14.5 ounces) diced tomatoes
- 4 cups low-sodium vegetable broth
- 1 teaspoon ground cumin
- 1 teaspoon ground coriander
- 1/2 teaspoon ground turmeric
- 1/4 teaspoon cayenne pepper (optional)
- 1 tablespoon lemon juice
- Fresh cilantro for garnish

Instructions

1. Heat the olive oil in a large pot over medium heat. Add the onion, garlic, carrots, and celery, and sauté until softened, about 5 minutes.
2. Stir in the ground cumin, ground coriander, ground turmeric, and cayenne pepper (if using). Cook for 1 minute.
3. Add the diced tomatoes, vegetable broth, and lentils. Bring to a boil, then reduce the heat and simmer for 30 minutes until the lentils are tender.
4. Stir in the lemon juice.
5. Garnish with fresh cilantro and serve immediately.

Nutrition Info (per serving)

- Calories: 250
- Protein: 12g
- Carbohydrates: 38g
- Fat: 7g
- Fiber: 15g
- Sugars: 9g
- Sodium: 250mg

3. Miso Soup with Tofu and Seaweed

Servings: 4

Cooking Time: 15 minutes

Ingredients

- 4 cups water
- 4 tablespoons miso paste
- 1 cup silken tofu, diced
- 1/4 cup dried seaweed (wakame)
- 2 green onions, sliced
- 1 tablespoon low-sodium soy sauce
- 1 teaspoon grated fresh ginger

Instructions

1. In a large pot, bring the water to a simmer over medium heat.
2. In a small bowl, mix the miso paste with a little hot water to dissolve. Add the dissolved miso to the pot.
3. Add the diced tofu, dried seaweed, soy sauce, and grated fresh ginger to the pot. Simmer for 5 minutes.
4. Stir in the sliced green onions.
5. Serve immediately.

Nutrition Info (per serving)

- Calories: 80
- Protein: 6g
- Carbohydrates: 8g
- Fat: 3g
- Fiber: 2g
- Sugars: 1g
- Sodium: 380mg

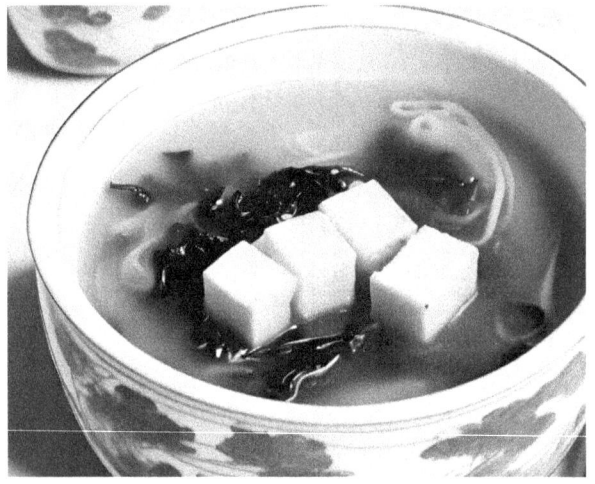

4. Turmeric Chicken Soup

Servings: 4
Cooking Time: 45 minutes
Ingredients

- 1 pound boneless, skinless chicken breasts, cut into bite-sized pieces
- 2 tablespoons olive oil
- 1 onion, chopped
- 3 garlic cloves, minced
- 1 tablespoon grated fresh ginger
- 2 carrots, sliced
- 2 celery stalks, sliced
- 4 cups low-sodium chicken broth
- 1 cup coconut milk (light)
- 1 teaspoon ground turmeric
- 1/2 teaspoon ground black pepper
- 1/2 teaspoon ground cumin
- 2 cups baby spinach
- 1 tablespoon lemon juice
- Fresh cilantro for garnish

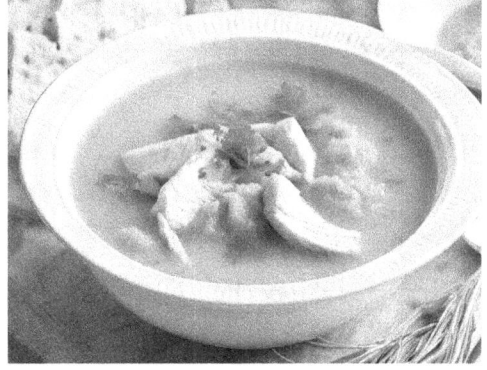

Instructions

1. Heat the olive oil in a large pot over medium heat. Add the chicken and cook until browned, about 5-7 minutes. Remove from the pot and set aside.
2. In the same pot, add the onion, garlic, and grated ginger, and sauté until softened, about 5 minutes.
3. Stir in the ground turmeric, ground black pepper, and ground cumin. Cook for 1 minute.
4. Add the carrots, celery, chicken broth, and coconut milk. Bring to a simmer.
5. Return the chicken to the pot and cook for 20 minutes until the chicken is cooked through and the vegetables are tender.
6. Stir in the baby spinach and lemon juice. Cook for another 2 minutes until the spinach is wilted.
7. Garnish with fresh cilantro and serve immediately.

Nutrition Info (per serving)

- Calories: 300
- Protein: 28g
- Carbohydrates: 16g
- Fat: 14g
- Fiber: 4g
- Sugars: 6g
- Sodium: 320mg

5. White Bean and Escarole Soup

Servings: 4

Cooking Time: 40 minutes

Ingredients

- 2 tablespoons olive oil
- 1 onion, chopped
- 3 garlic cloves, minced
- 2 carrots, diced
- 2 celery stalks, diced
- 1 can (14.5 ounces) white beans, rinsed and drained
- 4 cups low-sodium vegetable broth
- 4 cups chopped escarole
- 1 teaspoon dried thyme
- 1 tablespoon lemon juice
- Fresh parsley for garnish

Instructions

1. Heat the olive oil in a large pot over medium heat. Add the onion, garlic, carrots, and celery, and sauté until softened, about 5 minutes.
2. Stir in the white beans, vegetable broth, and dried thyme. Bring to a simmer and cook for 20 minutes.
3. Add the chopped escarole and cook for another 10 minutes until the escarole is tender.
4. Stir in the lemon juice.
5. Garnish with fresh parsley and serve immediately.

Nutrition Info (per serving)

- Calories: 250
- Protein: 10g
- Carbohydrates: 30g
- Fat: 10g
- Fiber: 8g
- Sugars: 7g
- Sodium: 250mg

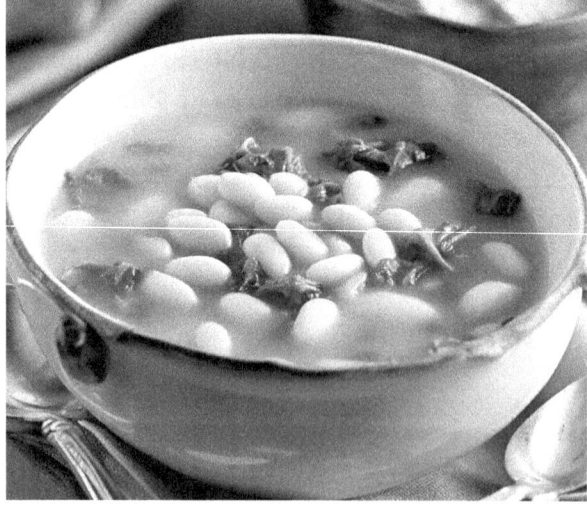

6. Spicy Black Bean Soup

Servings: 4
Cooking Time: 40 minutes

Ingredients

- 2 tablespoons olive oil
- 1 onion, chopped
- 3 garlic cloves, minced
- 2 carrots, diced
- 2 celery stalks, diced
- 1 red bell pepper, diced
- 2 cans (14.5 ounces each) black beans, rinsed and drained
- 4 cups low-sodium vegetable broth
- 1 teaspoon ground cumin
- 1 teaspoon smoked paprika
- 1/4 teaspoon cayenne pepper (optional)
- 1 tablespoon lime juice
- Fresh cilantro for garnish

Instructions

1. Heat the olive oil in a large pot over medium heat. Add the onion, garlic, carrots, celery, and red bell pepper, and sauté until softened, about 5 minutes.
2. Stir in the black beans, vegetable broth, ground cumin, smoked paprika, and cayenne pepper (if using). Bring to a simmer and cook for 25 minutes.
3. Use an immersion blender to blend the soup until smooth, or blend in batches using a regular blender.
4. Stir in the lime juice.
5. Garnish with fresh cilantro and serve immediately.

Nutrition Info (per serving)

- Calories: 280
- Protein: 14g
- Carbohydrates: 45g
- Fat: 7g
- Fiber: 15g
- Sugars: 6g
- Sodium: 280mg

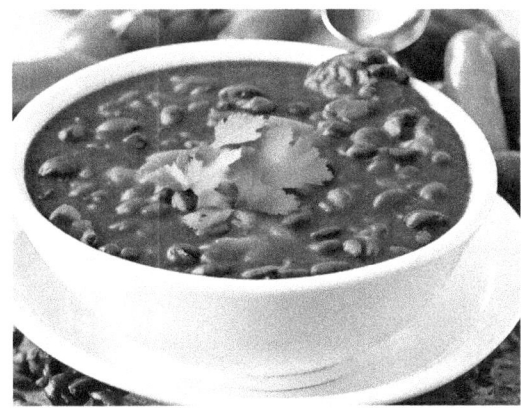

7. Sweet Potato and Coconut Soup
Servings: 4
Cooking Time: 35 minutes
Ingredients

- 2 tablespoons olive oil
- 1 onion, chopped
- 3 garlic cloves, minced
- 1 tablespoon grated fresh ginger
- 4 cups diced sweet potatoes
- 4 cups low-sodium vegetable broth
- 1 can (14 ounces) light coconut milk
- 1 teaspoon ground turmeric
- 1/2 teaspoon ground cinnamon
- 1/4 teaspoon cayenne pepper (optional)
- 1 tablespoon lime juice
- Fresh cilantro for garnish

Instructions

1. Heat the olive oil in a large pot over medium heat. Add the onion, garlic, and grated ginger, and sauté until softened, about 5 minutes.
2. Stir in the diced sweet potatoes, vegetable broth, coconut milk, ground turmeric, ground cinnamon, and cayenne pepper (if using). Bring to a simmer and cook for 20 minutes until the sweet potatoes are tender.
3. Use an immersion blender to blend the soup until smooth, or blend in batches using a regular blender.
4. Stir in the lime juice.
5. Garnish with fresh cilantro and serve immediately.

Nutrition Info (per serving)

- Calories: 320
- Protein: 4g
- Carbohydrates: 45g
- Fat: 14g
- Fiber: 7g
- Sugars: 12g
- Sodium: 300mg

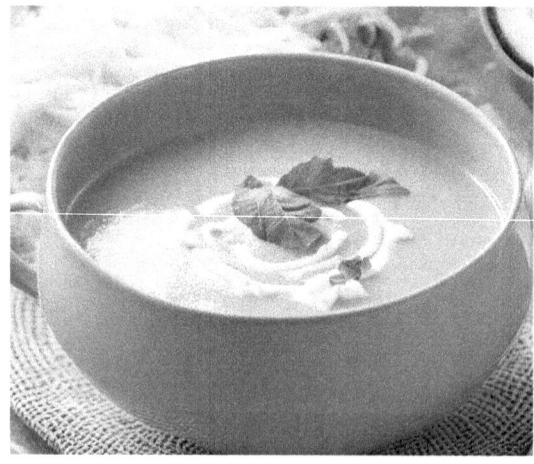

8. Salmon Chowder

Servings: 4
Cooking Time: 35 minutes
Ingredients

- 2 tablespoons olive oil
- 1 onion, chopped
- 3 garlic cloves, minced
- 2 celery stalks, diced
- 2 carrots, diced
- 2 potatoes, peeled and diced
- 4 cups low-sodium vegetable broth
- 1 cup light coconut milk
- 1 pound salmon fillet, skin removed and cut into bite-sized pieces
- 1 teaspoon dried thyme
- 1 tablespoon lemon juice
- Fresh dill for garnish

Instructions

1. Heat the olive oil in a large pot over medium heat. Add the onion, garlic, celery, and carrots, and sauté until softened, about 5 minutes.
2. Stir in the diced potatoes, vegetable broth, and dried thyme. Bring to a simmer and cook for 15 minutes until the potatoes are tender.
3. Add the coconut milk and salmon pieces. Cook for another 7-10 minutes until the salmon is cooked through.
4. Stir in the lemon juice.
5. Garnish with fresh dill and serve immediately.

Nutrition Info (per serving)

- Calories: 350
- Protein: 28g
- Carbohydrates: 30g
- Fat: 14g
- Fiber: 6g
- Sugars: 6g
- Sodium: 320mg

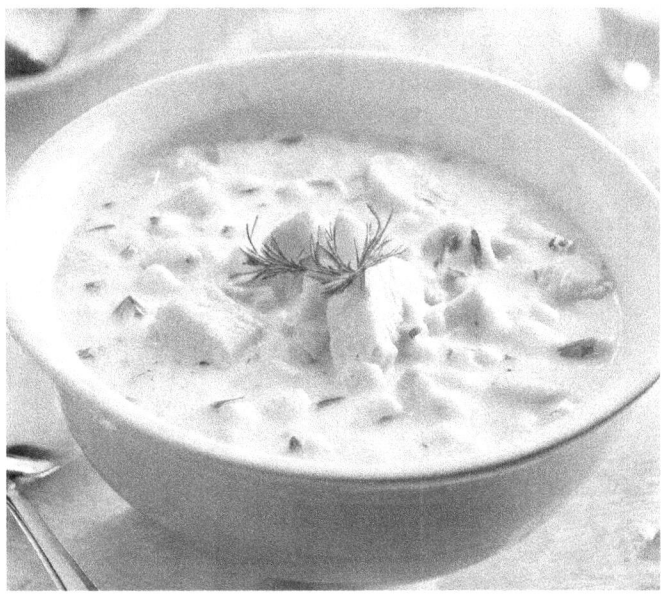

9. French Onion Soup

Servings: 4
Cooking Time: 1 hour

Ingredients

- 4 large onions, thinly sliced
- 3 tablespoons olive oil
- 1 teaspoon dried thyme
- 4 cups low-sodium vegetable broth
- 1 cup dry white wine (optional)
- 1 tablespoon balsamic vinegar
- 4 slices whole grain bread
- 1 cup grated Gruyere cheese

Instructions

1. Heat the olive oil in a large pot over medium heat. Add the sliced onions and cook, stirring occasionally, until they are caramelized, about 30 minutes.
2. Stir in the dried thyme, vegetable broth, white wine (if using), and balsamic vinegar. Bring to a simmer and cook for another 20 minutes.
3. Preheat the oven to 400°F (200°C). Place the slices of whole grain bread on a baking sheet and toast in the oven for 5 minutes.
4. Ladle the soup into oven-safe bowls. Place a slice of toasted bread on top of each bowl and sprinkle with grated Gruyere cheese.
5. Place the bowls on the baking sheet and broil in the oven for 3-5 minutes until the cheese is melted and bubbly.
6. Serve immediately.

Nutrition Info (per serving)

- Calories: 400
- Protein: 15g
- Carbohydrates: 50g
- Fat: 15g
- Fiber: 7g
- Sugars: 15g
- Sodium: 360mg

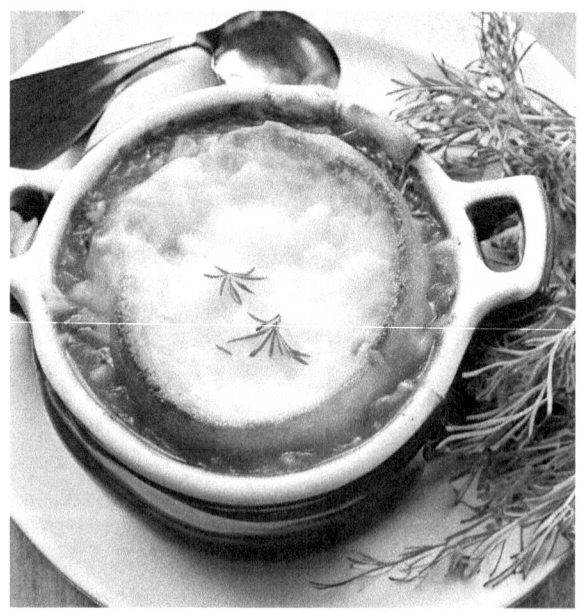

10. Tom Yum Soup

Servings: 4
Cooking Time: 30 minutes
Ingredients

- 4 cups low-sodium chicken broth
- 1 cup water
- 2 stalks lemongrass, cut into 2-inch pieces and smashed
- 3 slices galangal (or ginger)
- 3 kaffir lime leaves, torn
- 2 garlic cloves, minced
- 1 cup mushrooms, sliced
- 1 cup shrimp, peeled and deveined
- 2 tablespoons fish sauce
- 2 tablespoons lime juice
- 1 tablespoon Thai red curry paste
- 1/2 cup cherry tomatoes, halved
- Fresh cilantro for garnish

Instructions

1. In a large pot, combine the chicken broth, water, lemongrass, galangal (or ginger), kaffir lime leaves, and minced garlic. Bring to a boil, then reduce the heat and simmer for 10 minutes.
2. Add the sliced mushrooms and cook for another 5 minutes.
3. Stir in the shrimp, fish sauce, lime juice, and Thai red curry paste. Cook for another 5 minutes until the shrimp are pink and opaque.
4. Add the cherry tomatoes and cook for 2 more minutes.
5. Remove the lemongrass, galangal, and lime leaves before serving.
6. Garnish with fresh cilantro and serve immediately.

Nutrition Info (per serving)

- Calories: 200
- Protein: 20g
- Carbohydrates: 10g
- Fat: 8g
- Fiber: 2g
- Sugars: 4g
- Sodium: 450mg

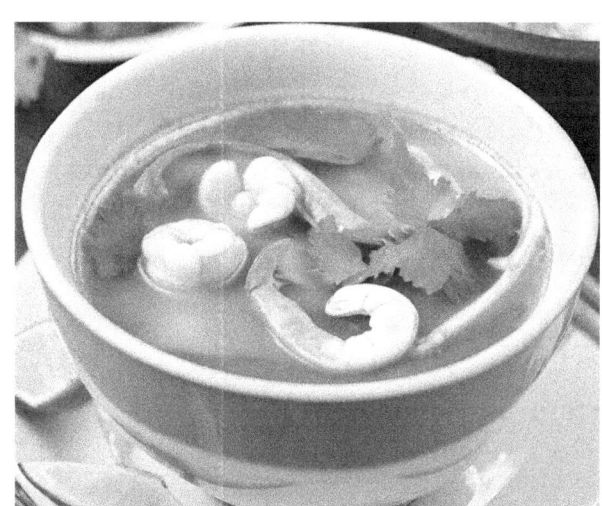

11. Italian Wedding Soup

Servings: 4
Cooking Time: 40 minutes
Ingredients
Meatballs:

- 1/2 pound ground turkey
- 1/4 cup whole grain breadcrumbs
- 1 egg, beaten
- 1/4 cup grated Parmesan cheese
- 1 garlic clove, minced
- 1 teaspoon dried oregano

Soup:

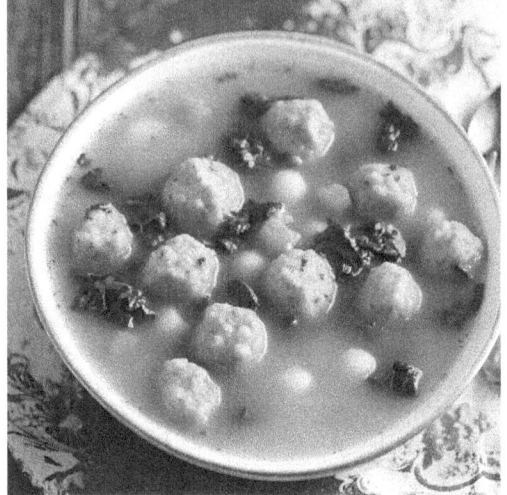

- 2 tablespoons olive oil
- 1 onion, chopped
- 2 garlic cloves, minced
- 2 carrots, sliced
- 2 celery stalks, sliced
- 6 cups low-sodium chicken broth
- 1/2 cup uncooked whole grain pasta (orzo or small shells)
- 4 cups fresh spinach, chopped
- 1 tablespoon lemon juice
- Fresh parsley for garnish

Instructions

1. For the Meatballs: In a large bowl, combine the ground turkey, breadcrumbs, beaten egg, Parmesan cheese, minced garlic, and dried oregano. Mix well and form into small meatballs.
2. Heat 1 tablespoon of olive oil in a large pot over medium heat. Add the meatballs and cook until browned on all sides, about 5-7 minutes. Remove from the pot and set aside.
3. For the Soup: In the same pot, add the remaining tablespoon of olive oil. Add the onion, garlic, carrots, and celery. Sauté until softened, about 5 minutes.
4. Stir in the chicken broth and bring to a simmer.
5. Add the pasta and cook for about 10 minutes until the pasta is tender.
6. Return the meatballs to the pot and add the chopped spinach. Cook for another 5 minutes until the spinach is wilted.
7. Stir in the lemon juice.
8. Garnish with fresh parsley and serve immediately.

Nutrition Info (per serving)
Calories: 320   Protein: 28g   Carbohydrates: 30g   Fat: 12g   Fiber: 6g

- Sugars: 7g
- Sodium: 380mg

12. Kale and White Bean Soup
Servings: 4
Cooking Time: 35 minutes
Ingredients

- 2 tablespoons olive oil
- 1 onion, chopped
- 3 garlic cloves, minced
- 2 carrots, diced
- 2 celery stalks, diced
- 4 cups chopped kale, stems removed
- 1 can (14.5 ounces) white beans, rinsed and drained
- 4 cups low-sodium vegetable broth
- 1 teaspoon dried thyme
- 1 teaspoon dried rosemary
- 1 tablespoon lemon juice
- Fresh parsley for garnish

Instructions

1. Heat the olive oil in a large pot over medium heat. Add the onion, garlic, carrots, and celery, and sauté until softened, about 5 minutes.
2. Stir in the chopped kale and cook for another 3 minutes until wilted.
3. Add the white beans, vegetable broth, dried thyme, and dried rosemary. Bring to a simmer and cook for 20 minutes.
4. Stir in the lemon juice.
5. Garnish with fresh parsley and serve immediately.

Nutrition Info (per serving)

- Calories: 250
- Protein: 10g
- Carbohydrates: 35g
- Fat: 8g
- Fiber: 9g
- Sugars: 7g
- Sodium: 260mg

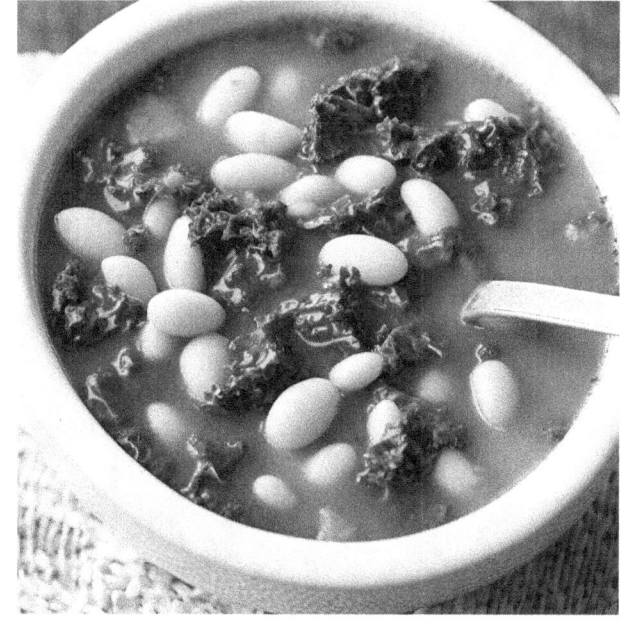

13. Seafood Stew

Servings: 4
Cooking Time: 40 minutes
Ingredients

- 2 tablespoons olive oil
- 1 onion, chopped
- 3 garlic cloves, minced
- 1 fennel bulb, thinly sliced
- 1 red bell pepper, diced
- 1 can (14.5 ounces) diced tomatoes
- 4 cups low-sodium vegetable broth
- 1/2 cup dry white wine (optional)
- 1 teaspoon dried thyme
- 1/2 teaspoon dried oregano
- 1/2 teaspoon paprika
- 1 pound firm white fish (cod, halibut), cut into chunks
- 1/2 pound shrimp, peeled and deveined
- 1/2 pound mussels, scrubbed and debearded
- 1/4 cup fresh parsley, chopped
- 1 tablespoon lemon juice

Instructions

1. Heat the olive oil in a large pot over medium heat. Add the onion, garlic, fennel, and red bell pepper. Sauté until softened, about 5 minutes.
2. Stir in the diced tomatoes, vegetable broth, white wine (if using), dried thyme, oregano, and paprika. Bring to a simmer and cook for 15 minutes.
3. Add the fish, shrimp, and mussels. Cover and cook for another 7-10 minutes until the seafood is cooked through and the mussels have opened.
4. Stir in the lemon juice and garnish with fresh parsley.
5. Serve immediately.

Nutrition Info (per serving)

- Calories: 320
- Protein: 30g
- Carbohydrates: 18g
- Fat: 12g
- Fiber: 4g
- Sugars: 7g
- Sodium: 450mg

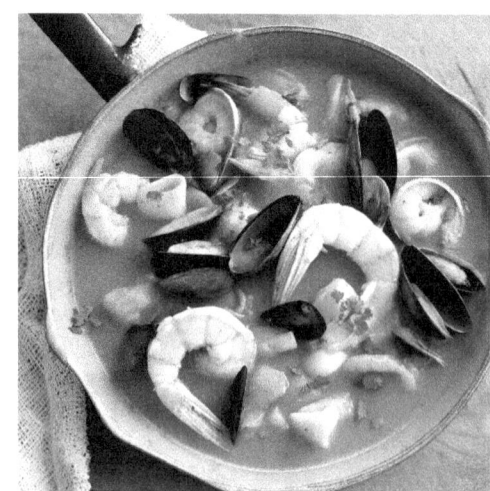

14. Gazpacho
Servings: 4
Cooking Time: 15 minutes (plus chilling time)
Ingredients

- 6 ripe tomatoes, chopped
- 1 cucumber, peeled and chopped
- 1 red bell pepper, chopped
- 1 green bell pepper, chopped
- 1 small red onion, chopped
- 3 garlic cloves, minced
- 1/4 cup olive oil
- 2 tablespoons red wine vinegar
- 2 cups low-sodium vegetable broth
- 1 teaspoon ground cumin
- 1/4 teaspoon cayenne pepper (optional)
- Fresh basil for garnish

Instructions

1. In a blender or food processor, combine the tomatoes, cucumber, red bell pepper, green bell pepper, red onion, garlic, olive oil, red wine vinegar, vegetable broth, ground cumin, and cayenne pepper (if using).
2. Blend until smooth.
3. Chill the soup in the refrigerator for at least 2 hours before serving.
4. Garnish with fresh basil and serve cold.

Nutrition Info (per serving)

- Calories: 180
- Protein: 3g
- Carbohydrates: 18g
- Fat: 12g
- Fiber: 4g
- Sugars: 10g
- Sodium: 200mg

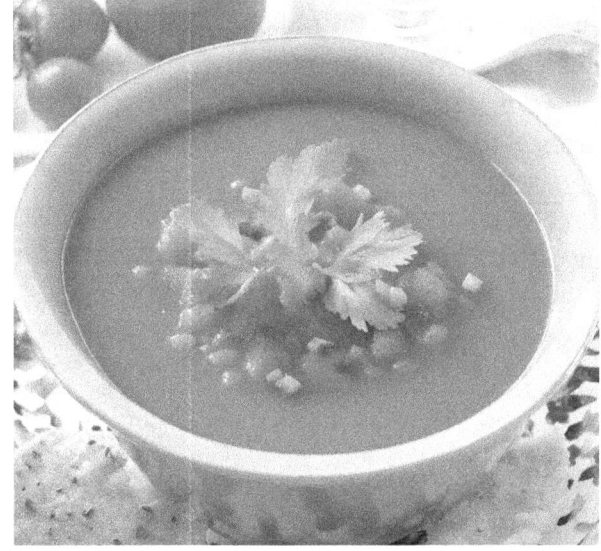

15. Chicken and Wild Rice Soup

Servings: 4

Cooking Time: 50 minutes

Ingredients

- 2 tablespoons olive oil
- 1 onion, chopped
- 3 garlic cloves, minced
- 2 carrots, diced
- 2 celery stalks, diced
- 1 cup wild rice, rinsed
- 6 cups low-sodium chicken broth
- 1 pound boneless, skinless chicken breasts, cut into bite-sized pieces
- 1 teaspoon dried thyme
- 1 teaspoon dried rosemary
- 1/2 cup light coconut milk
- 1 tablespoon lemon juice
- Fresh parsley for garnish

Instructions

1. Heat the olive oil in a large pot over medium heat. Add the onion, garlic, carrots, and celery. Sauté until softened, about 5 minutes.
2. Stir in the wild rice and cook for 1 minute.
3. Add the chicken broth, chicken pieces, dried thyme, and rosemary. Bring to a simmer and cook for 40 minutes until the rice is tender and the chicken is cooked through.
4. Stir in the light coconut milk and lemon juice.
5. Garnish with fresh parsley and serve immediately.

Nutrition Info (per serving)

- Calories: 340
- Protein: 28g
- Carbohydrates: 35g
- Fat: 12g
- Fiber: 5g
- Sugars: 4g
- Sodium: 350mg

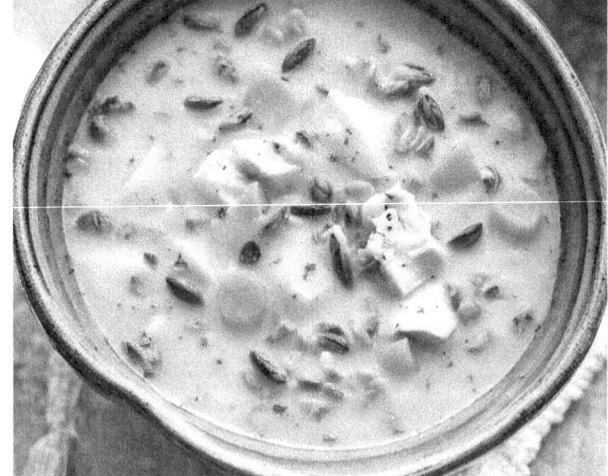

16. Potato Leek Soup

Servings: 4
Cooking Time: 35 minutes
Ingredients

- 2 tablespoons olive oil
- 3 leeks, white and light green parts only, sliced
- 3 garlic cloves, minced
- 4 potatoes, peeled and diced
- 4 cups low-sodium vegetable broth
- 1 cup light coconut milk
- 1 teaspoon dried thyme
- 1 tablespoon lemon juice
- Fresh chives for garnish

Instructions

1. Heat the olive oil in a large pot over medium heat. Add the leeks and garlic. Sauté until softened, about 5 minutes.
2. Stir in the potatoes, vegetable broth, dried thyme, and coconut milk. Bring to a simmer and cook for 25 minutes until the potatoes are tender.
3. Use an immersion blender to blend the soup until smooth, or blend in batches using a regular blender.
4. Stir in the lemon juice.
5. Garnish with fresh chives and serve immediately.

Nutrition Info (per serving)

- Calories: 280
- Protein: 5g
- Carbohydrates: 45g
- Fat: 10g
- Fiber: 6g
- Sugars: 4g
- Sodium: 300mg

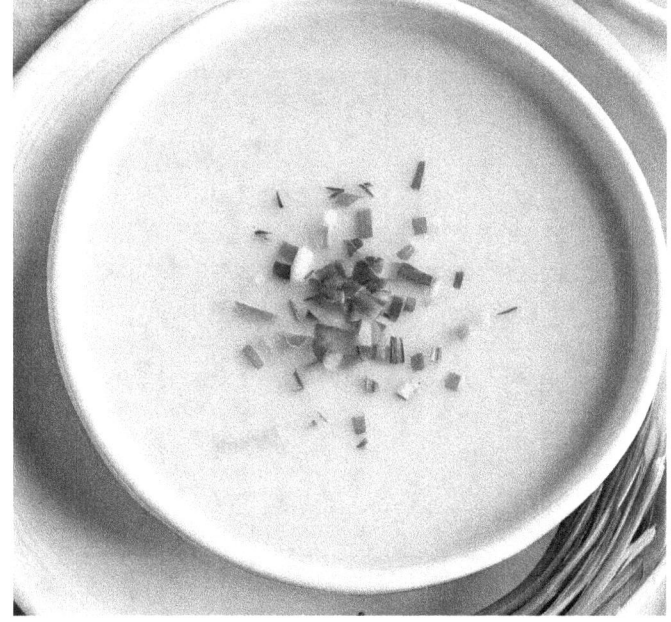

17. Vegetable Lentil Stew
Servings: 4
Cooking Time: 45 minutes
Ingredients

- 2 tablespoons olive oil
- 1 onion, chopped
- 3 garlic cloves, minced
- 2 carrots, diced
- 2 celery stalks, diced
- 1 red bell pepper, diced
- 1 cup dried lentils, rinsed
- 4 cups low-sodium vegetable broth
- 1 can (14.5 ounces) diced tomatoes
- 1 teaspoon ground cumin
- 1 teaspoon ground coriander
- 1/2 teaspoon smoked paprika
- 1 tablespoon lemon juice
- Fresh cilantro for garnish

Instructions

1. Heat the olive oil in a large pot over medium heat. Add the onion, garlic, carrots, celery, and red bell pepper. Sauté until softened, about 5 minutes.
2. Stir in the lentils, vegetable broth, diced tomatoes, ground cumin, ground coriander, and smoked paprika. Bring to a simmer and cook for 30 minutes until the lentils are tender.
3. Stir in the lemon juice.
4. Garnish with fresh cilantro and serve immediately.

Nutrition Info (per serving)

- Calories: 300
- Protein: 14g
- Carbohydrates: 45g
- Fat: 8g
- Fiber: 15g
- Sugars: 10g
- Sodium: 280mg

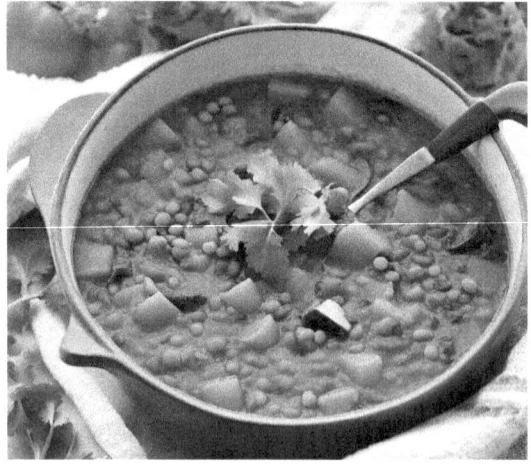

18. Zucchini Basil Soup

Servings: 4
Cooking Time: 30 minutes
Ingredients

- 2 tablespoons olive oil
- 1 onion, chopped
- 3 garlic cloves, minced
- 4 zucchini, chopped
- 4 cups low-sodium vegetable broth
- 1 cup light coconut milk
- 1 cup fresh basil leaves
- 1 tablespoon lemon juice

Instructions

1. Heat the olive oil in a large pot over medium heat. Add the onion and garlic. Sauté until softened, about 5 minutes.
2. Stir in the chopped zucchini and cook for another 5 minutes.
3. Add the vegetable broth and bring to a simmer. Cook for 15 minutes until the zucchini is tender.
4. Use an immersion blender to blend the soup until smooth, or blend in batches using a regular blender.
5. Stir in the coconut milk and fresh basil leaves.
6. Add the lemon juice and blend again until smooth.
7. Serve immediately.

Nutrition Info (per serving)

- Calories: 220
- Protein: 4g
- Carbohydrates: 20g
- Fat: 15g
- Fiber: 4g
- Sugars: 10g
- Sodium: 240mg

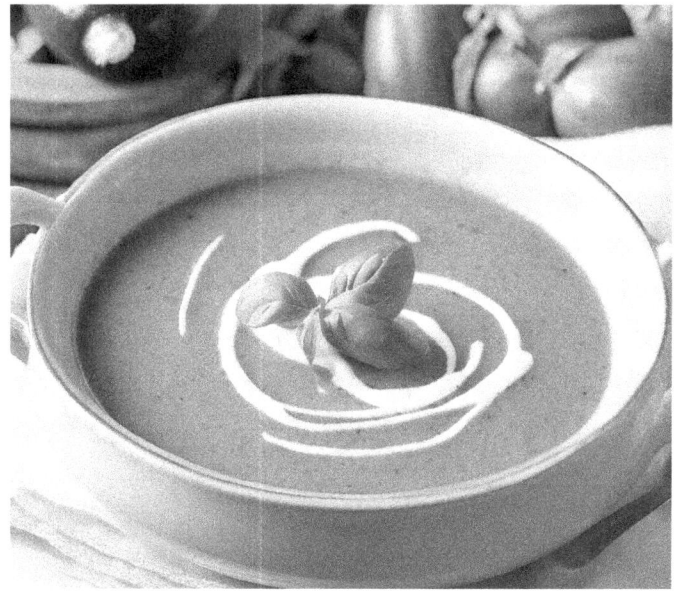

19. Pea and Ham Hock Soup

Servings: 4
Cooking Time: 1 hour 30 minutes
Ingredients

- 1 ham hock
- 2 tablespoons olive oil
- 1 onion, chopped
- 3 garlic cloves, minced
- 2 carrots, diced
- 2 celery stalks, diced
- 4 cups low-sodium chicken broth
- 2 cups water
- 2 cups frozen peas
- 1 teaspoon dried thyme
- 1 tablespoon lemon juice
- Fresh mint for garnish

Instructions

1. In a large pot, combine the ham hock, chicken broth, and water. Bring to a simmer and cook for 1 hour until the ham is tender.
2. Remove the ham hock from the pot, let cool, and shred the meat.
3. In a separate skillet, heat the olive oil over medium heat. Add the onion, garlic, carrots, and celery. Sauté until softened, about 5 minutes.
4. Add the sautéed vegetables to the pot with the broth. Stir in the frozen peas and dried thyme. Bring to a simmer and cook for 15 minutes.
5. Return the shredded ham to the pot and stir in the lemon juice.
6. Garnish with fresh mint and serve immediately.

Nutrition Info (per serving)

- Calories: 300
- Protein: 20g
- Carbohydrates: 28g
- Fat: 12g
- Fiber: 7g
- Sugars: 10g
- Sodium: 450mg

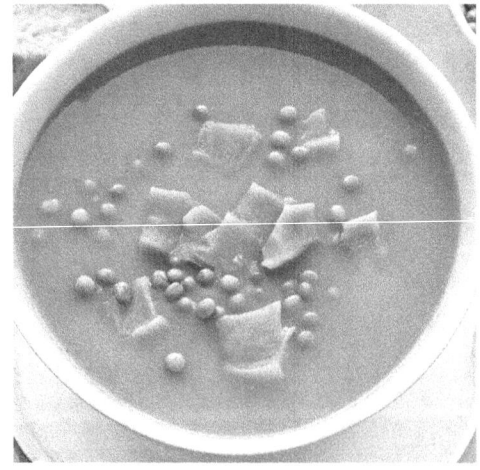

10-WEEK MEAL PLAN

Week 1
Monday
- Breakfast: Baked Avocado Eggs
- Lunch: Grilled Chicken with Avocado Salsa
- Dinner: Chicken and Kale Stew
- Snack: Apple Cinnamon Porridge

Tuesday
- Breakfast: Avocado and Egg Breakfast Pizza
- Lunch: Shrimp and Mango Salad
- Dinner: Lentil Tomato Soup
- Snack: Greek Yogurt Parfait

Wednesday
- Breakfast: Pomegranate and Pistachio Porridge
- Lunch: Spinach and Avocado Wrap
- Dinner: Turmeric Chicken Soup
- Snack: Cucumber and Mint Smoothie

Thursday
- Breakfast: Pear and Gorgonzola Salad
- Lunch: Tuna Nicoise Salad
- Dinner: White Bean and Escarole Soup
- Snack: Whole Grain Waffles with Blueberry Compote

Friday
- Breakfast: Whole Grain Waffles with Blueberry Compote
- Lunch: Walnut and Banana Smoothie
- Dinner: Chicken and Sweet Potato Stew
- Snack: Zucchini Bread

Saturday
- Breakfast: Apple Cinnamon Porridge
- Lunch: Balsamic Glazed Chicken
- Dinner: Miso Soup with Tofu and Seaweed
- Snack: Kiwi and Strawberry Salad

Sunday
- Breakfast: Savory Oatmeal with Tomato and Spinach
- Lunch: Mediterranean Chicken and Grain Bowl
- Dinner: Seafood Stew
- Snack: Carrot and Apple Muffins

Week 2

Monday
- Breakfast: Egg and Quinoa Breakfast Cups
- Lunch: Chicken Gyros with Tzatziki
- Dinner: Chicken and Wild Rice Soup
- Snack: Broccoli and Cheese Oatmeal

Tuesday
- Breakfast: Banana Pancakes
- Lunch: Lemon and Rosemary Roast Chicken
- Dinner: Spicy Black Bean Soup
- Snack: Peach and Raspberry Smoothie

Wednesday
- Breakfast: Cottage Cheese with Pineapple and Chia Seeds
- Lunch: Sesame Chicken Salad
- Dinner: Sweet Potato and Coconut Soup
- Snack: Vegetable Hash with Poached Egg

Thursday
- Breakfast: Savory Oatmeal with Tomato and Spinach
- Lunch: Pesto Grilled Shrimp
- Dinner: Salmon Chowder
- Snack: Baked Pear with Honey and Walnuts

Friday
- Breakfast: Overnight Oats with Mango
- Lunch: Greek Chicken Salad
- Dinner: Potato Leek Soup
- Snack: Spinach and Feta Stuffed Chicken

Saturday
- Breakfast: Walnut and Banana Smoothie
- Lunch: Chicken Stir Fry with Broccoli and Ginger
- Dinner: French Onion Soup
- Snack: Turkey Chili

Sunday
- Breakfast: Apple Cinnamon Porridge
- Lunch: Zucchini Basil Soup
- Dinner: Pea and Ham Hock Soup
- Snack: Mushroom and Spinach Toast

Week 3

Monday
- Breakfast: Kiwi and Strawberry Salad
- Lunch: Herb-Roasted Turkey Breast
- Dinner: Vegetable Lentil Stew
- Snack: Tofu Scramble

Tuesday
- Breakfast: Egg and Quinoa Breakfast Cups
- Lunch: Turkey and Spinach Meatloaf
- Dinner: Italian Wedding Soup
- Snack: Tuna Nicoise Salad

Wednesday
- Breakfast: Baked Avocado Eggs
- Lunch: Spiced Chicken with Couscous
- Dinner: Grilled Mackerel with Herb Salad
- Snack: Carrot and Apple Muffins

Thursday
- Breakfast: Greek Yogurt Parfait
- Lunch: Lemon Garlic Chicken Thighs
- Dinner: Gazpacho
- Snack: Pear and Gorgonzola Salad

Friday
- Breakfast: Apple Cinnamon Porridge
- Lunch: Buffalo Chicken Salad
- Dinner: Thai Chicken Curry
- Snack: Zucchini Bread

Saturday
- Breakfast: Pomegranate and Pistachio Porridge
- Lunch: Chicken Paprikash
- Dinner: Tom Yum Soup
- Snack: Savory Oatmeal with Tomato and Spinach

Sunday
- Breakfast: Whole Grain Waffles with Blueberry Compote
- Lunch: Turkey Bolognese
- Dinner: Chicken and Kale Stew
- Snack: Shrimp and Mango Salad

Week 4

Monday
- Breakfast: Banana Pancakes
- Lunch: Pesto Chicken Bake
- Dinner: Lentil Tomato Soup
- Snack: Balsamic Glazed Chicken

Tuesday
- Breakfast: Cottage Cheese with Pineapple and Chia Seeds
- Lunch: Grilled Swordfish with Mango Salsa
- Dinner: Turmeric Chicken Soup
- Snack: Spinach and Feta Stuffed Chicken

Wednesday
- Breakfast: Kiwi and Strawberry Salad
- Lunch: Chicken Gyros with Tzatziki
- Dinner: White Bean and Escarole Soup
- Snack: Vegetable Hash with Poached Egg

Thursday
- Breakfast: Walnut and Banana Smoothie
- Lunch: Seafood Paella
- Dinner: Spicy Black Bean Soup
- Snack: Tuna Nicoise Salad

Friday
- Breakfast: Apple Cinnamon Porridge
- Lunch: Moroccan Chicken Tagine
- Dinner: Sweet Potato and Coconut Soup
- Snack: Cucumber and Mint Smoothie

Saturday
- Breakfast: Greek Yogurt Parfait
- Lunch: Grilled Chicken with Avocado Salsa
- Dinner: Salmon Chowder
- Snack: Pear and Gorgonzola Salad

Sunday
- Breakfast: Egg and Quinoa Breakfast Cups
- Lunch: Lemon and Rosemary Roast Chicken
- Dinner: Potato Leek Soup
- Snack: Baked Pear with Honey and Walnuts

Week 5

Monday
- Breakfast: Baked Avocado Eggs
- Lunch: Turkey Chili
- Dinner: French Onion Soup
- Snack: Mushroom and Spinach Toast

Tuesday
- Breakfast: Avocado and Egg Breakfast Pizza
- Lunch: Turkey and Spinach Meatloaf
- Dinner: Vegetable Lentil Stew
- Snack: Pomegranate and Pistachio Porridge

Wednesday
- Breakfast: Pear and Gorgonzola Salad
- Lunch: Buffalo Chicken Salad
- Dinner: Gazpacho
- Snack: Greek Yogurt Parfait

Thursday
- Breakfast: Kiwi and Strawberry Salad
- Lunch: Lemon Garlic Chicken Thighs
- Dinner: Tom Yum Soup
- Snack: Savory Oatmeal with Tomato and Spinach

Friday
- Breakfast: Whole Grain Waffles with Blueberry Compote
- Lunch: Sesame Chicken Salad
- Dinner: Thai Chicken Curry
- Snack: Walnut and Banana Smoothie

Saturday
- Breakfast: Cottage Cheese with Pineapple and Chia Seeds
- Lunch: Spiced Chicken with Couscous
- Dinner: Italian Wedding Soup
- Snack: Apple Cinnamon Porridge

Sunday
- Breakfast: Egg and Quinoa Breakfast Cups
- Lunch: Herb-Roasted Turkey Breast
- Dinner: Seafood Stew
- Snack: Tuna Nicoise Salad

Week 6

Monday
- Breakfast: Tofu Scramble
- Lunch: Salmon and Spinach Quiche
- Dinner: Zucchini Basil Soup
- Snack: Carrot and Apple Muffins

Tuesday
- Breakfast: Overnight Oats with Mango
- Lunch: Chicken and Quinoa Salad
- Dinner: Balsamic Glazed Chicken
- Snack: Greek Yogurt Parfait

Wednesday
- Breakfast: Apple Cinnamon Porridge
- Lunch: Herb-Roasted Turkey Breast
- Dinner: Turmeric Chicken Soup
- Snack: Spinach and Avocado Wrap

Thursday
- Breakfast: Whole Grain Waffles with Blueberry Compote
- Lunch: Turkey Bolognese
- Dinner: Lentil Tomato Soup
- Snack: Baked Pear with Honey and Walnuts

Friday
- Breakfast: Mushroom and Spinach Toast
- Lunch: Chicken Gyros with Tzatziki
- Dinner: Sweet Potato and Coconut Soup
- Snack: Kiwi and Strawberry Salad

Saturday
- Breakfast: Cottage Cheese with Pineapple and Chia Seeds
- Lunch: Moroccan Chicken Tagine
- Dinner: French Onion Soup
- Snack: Carrot and Apple Muffins

Sunday
- Breakfast: Banana Pancakes
- Lunch: Spiced Chicken with Couscous
- Dinner: Pea and Ham Hock Soup
- Snack: Greek Yogurt Parfait

Week 7

Monday
- Breakfast: Egg and Quinoa Breakfast Cups
- Lunch: Lemon and Rosemary Roast Chicken
- Dinner: Potato Leek Soup
- Snack: Savory Oatmeal with Tomato and Spinach

Tuesday
- Breakfast: Avocado and Egg Breakfast Pizza
- Lunch: Buffalo Chicken Salad
- Dinner: Seafood Stew
- Snack: Kiwi and Strawberry Salad

Wednesday
- Breakfast: Pear and Gorgonzola Salad
- Lunch: Mediterranean Chicken and Grain Bowl
- Dinner: Zucchini Basil Soup
- Snack: Walnut and Banana Smoothie

Thursday
- Breakfast: Greek Yogurt Parfait
- Lunch: Grilled Swordfish with Mango Salsa
- Dinner: Italian Wedding Soup
- Snack: Baked Pear with Honey and Walnuts

Friday
- Breakfast: Overnight Oats with Mango
- Lunch: Chicken and Wild Rice Soup
- Dinner: Tom Yum Soup
- Snack: Cucumber and Mint Smoothie

Saturday
- Breakfast: Tofu Scramble
- Lunch: Salmon Chowder
- Dinner: Vegetable Lentil Stew
- Snack: Apple Cinnamon Porridge

Sunday
- Breakfast: Whole Grain Waffles with Blueberry Compote
- Lunch: Turkey Chili
- Dinner: White Bean and Escarole Soup
- Snack: Greek Yogurt Parfait

Week 8

Monday
- Breakfast: Baked Avocado Eggs
- Lunch: Herb-Roasted Turkey Breast
- Dinner: Pea and Ham Hock Soup
- Snack: Carrot and Apple Muffins

Tuesday
- Breakfast: Apple Cinnamon Porridge
- Lunch: Pesto Chicken Bake
- Dinner: Seafood Stew
- Snack: Spinach and Avocado Wrap

Wednesday
- Breakfast: Banana Pancakes
- Lunch: Lemon Garlic Chicken Thighs
- Dinner: Turmeric Chicken Soup
- Snack: Kiwi and Strawberry Salad

Thursday
- Breakfast: Overnight Oats with Mango
- Lunch: Buffalo Chicken Salad
- Dinner: Lentil Tomato Soup
- Snack: Greek Yogurt Parfait

Friday
- Breakfast: Cottage Cheese with Pineapple and Chia Seeds
- Lunch: Chicken and Sweet Potato Stew
- Dinner: Zucchini Basil Soup
- Snack: Pear and Gorgonzola Salad

Saturday
- Breakfast: Whole Grain Waffles with Blueberry Compote
- Lunch: Sesame Chicken Salad
- Dinner: Potato Leek Soup
- Snack: Apple Cinnamon Porridge

Sunday
- Breakfast: Egg and Quinoa Breakfast Cups
- Lunch: Greek Chicken Salad
- Dinner: French Onion Soup
- Snack: Carrot and Apple Muffins

Week 9

Monday
- Breakfast: Greek Yogurt Parfait
- Lunch: Chicken Gyros with Tzatziki
- Dinner: Balsamic Glazed Chicken
- Snack: Kiwi and Strawberry Salad

Tuesday
- Breakfast: Mushroom and Spinach Toast
- Lunch: Grilled Chicken with Avocado Salsa
- Dinner: Pea and Ham Hock Soup
- Snack: Cucumber and Mint Smoothie

Wednesday
- Breakfast: Tofu Scramble
- Lunch: Spiced Chicken with Couscous
- Dinner: Seafood Stew
- Snack: Overnight Oats with Mango

Thursday
- Breakfast: Banana Pancakes
- Lunch: Lemon and Rosemary Roast Chicken
- Dinner: Tom Yum Soup
- Snack: Whole Grain Waffles with Blueberry Compote

Friday
- Breakfast: Egg and Quinoa Breakfast Cups
- Lunch: Mediterranean Chicken and Grain Bowl
- Dinner: White Bean and Escarole Soup
- Snack: Apple Cinnamon Porridge

Saturday
- Breakfast: Cottage Cheese with Pineapple and Chia Seeds
- Lunch: Salmon Chowder
- Dinner: Potato Leek Soup
- Snack: Carrot and Apple Muffins

Sunday
- Breakfast: Greek Yogurt Parfait
- Lunch: Buffalo Chicken Salad
- Dinner: Vegetable Lentil Stew
- Snack: Kiwi and Strawberry Salad

Week 10

Monday
- Breakfast: Whole Grain Waffles with Blueberry Compote
- Lunch: Herb-Roasted Turkey Breast
- Dinner: French Onion Soup
- Snack: Greek Yogurt Parfait

Tuesday
- Breakfast: Baked Avocado Eggs
- Lunch: Chicken Gyros with Tzatziki
- Dinner: Zucchini Basil Soup
- Snack: Apple Cinnamon Porridge

Wednesday
- Breakfast: Banana Pancakes
- Lunch: Pesto Chicken Bake
- Dinner: Turmeric Chicken Soup
- Snack: Carrot and Apple Muffins

Thursday
- Breakfast: Overnight Oats with Mango
- Lunch: Lemon Garlic Chicken Thighs
- Dinner: Tom Yum Soup
- Snack: Kiwi and Strawberry Salad

Friday
- Breakfast: Mushroom and Spinach Toast
- Lunch: Grilled Swordfish with Mango Salsa
- Dinner: Potato Leek Soup
- Snack: Greek Yogurt Parfait

Saturday
- Breakfast: Cottage Cheese with Pineapple and Chia Seeds
- Lunch: Chicken and Sweet Potato Stew
- Dinner: Lentil Tomato Soup
- Snack: Whole Grain Waffles with Blueberry Compote

Sunday
- Breakfast: Greek Yogurt Parfait
- Lunch: Mediterranean Chicken and Grain Bowl
- Dinner: Pea and Ham Hock Soup
- Snack: Apple Cinnamon Porridge

WEEKLY MEAL PLANNER + WORKBOOK

	BREAKFAST	LUNCH	DINNER	SNACKS
MONDAY				
TUESDAY				
WEDNESDAY				
THURSDAY				
FRIDAY				
SATURDAY				
SUNDAY				

What are your primary goals for following the Giant Cell Arteritis diet?
- Write down at least three specific health goals you aim to achieve with this diet.

....

....

....

....

....

....

WEEKLY MEAL PLANNER + WORKBOOK

	BREAKFAST	LUNCH	DINNER	SNACKS
MONDAY				
TUESDAY				
WEDNESDAY				
THURSDAY				
FRIDAY				
SATURDAY				
SUNDAY				

How do you currently feel about your eating habits?
- Reflect on your current diet and list any areas you feel need improvement.

....

....

....

....

....

....

WEEKLY MEAL PLANNER + WORKBOOK

	BREAKFAST	LUNCH	DINNER	SNACKS
MONDAY				
TUESDAY				
WEDNESDAY				
THURSDAY				
FRIDAY				
SATURDAY				
SUNDAY				

What challenges do you anticipate facing when starting this new diet?
- Identify potential obstacles and think of strategies to overcome them.

....

....

....

....

....

....

WEEKLY MEAL PLANNER + WORKBOOK

	BREAKFAST	LUNCH	DINNER	SNACKS
MONDAY				
TUESDAY				
WEDNESDAY				
THURSDAY				
FRIDAY				
SATURDAY				
SUNDAY				

- How can you incorporate more anti-inflammatory foods into your daily meals? List five anti-inflammatory foods you can easily add to your diet.

....

....

....

....

....

....

WEEKLY MEAL PLANNER + WORKBOOK

	BREAKFAST	LUNCH	DINNER	SNACKS
MONDAY				
TUESDAY				
WEDNESDAY				
THURSDAY				
FRIDAY				
SATURDAY				
SUNDAY				

Which foods should you avoid to manage Giant Cell Arteritis effectively?

- Make a list of foods known to exacerbate inflammation and plan alternatives.

....

....

....

....

....

....

WEEKLY MEAL PLANNER + WORKBOOK

	BREAKFAST	LUNCH	DINNER	SNACKS
MONDAY				
TUESDAY				
WEDNESDAY				
THURSDAY				
FRIDAY				
SATURDAY				
SUNDAY				

What are your favorite fruits and vegetables, and how can you include them in your diet?

- List your top five favorite fruits and vegetables and brainstorm meal ideas that incorporate them.

....

....

....

....

....

....

WEEKLY MEAL PLANNER + WORKBOOK

	BREAKFAST	LUNCH	DINNER	SNACKS
MONDAY				
TUESDAY				
WEDNESDAY				
THURSDAY				
FRIDAY				
SATURDAY				
SUNDAY				

Who can support you in your dietary changes, and how can you involve them?
- List family members, friends, or support groups that can help you stay accountable.

....

....

....

....

....

....

WEEKLY MEAL PLANNER + WORKBOOK

	BREAKFAST	LUNCH	DINNER	SNACKS
MONDAY				
TUESDAY				
WEDNESDAY				
THURSDAY				
FRIDAY				
SATURDAY				
SUNDAY				

What are some healthy substitutes for your favorite unhealthy foods?
- **Identify at least three unhealthy foods you enjoy and find healthier alternatives.**

....

....

....

....

....

....

WEEKLY MEAL PLANNER + WORKBOOK

	BREAKFAST	LUNCH	DINNER	SNACKS
MONDAY				
TUESDAY				
WEDNESDAY				
THURSDAY				
FRIDAY				
SATURDAY				
SUNDAY				

What steps can you take to reduce your sugar intake? List ways to cut down on added sugars in your diet and identify natural sweeteners you can use instead.

....

....

....

....

....

....

WEEKLY MEAL PLANNER + WORKBOOK

	BREAKFAST	LUNCH	DINNER	SNACKS
MONDAY				
TUESDAY				
WEDNESDAY				
THURSDAY				
FRIDAY				
SATURDAY				
SUNDAY				

- How will you handle social situations where unhealthy food is served?
  Plan strategies for navigating social events without compromising your diet.

....

....

....

....

....

....

WEEKLY MEAL PLANNER + WORKBOOK

	BREAKFAST	LUNCH	DINNER	SNACKS
MONDAY				
TUESDAY				
WEDNESDAY				
THURSDAY				
FRIDAY				
SATURDAY				
SUNDAY				

What are your favorite ways to cook and prepare meals? Describe your preferred cooking methods and how they can be adapted to fit the Giant Cell Arteritis diet.

....

....

....

....

....

....

WEEKLY MEAL PLANNER + WORKBOOK

	BREAKFAST	LUNCH	DINNER	SNACKS
MONDAY				
TUESDAY				
WEDNESDAY				
THURSDAY				
FRIDAY				
SATURDAY				
SUNDAY				

How can you add more fiber to your diet?
- Identify high-fiber foods and plan to include them in your daily meals.

....

....

....

....

....

....

WEEKLY MEAL PLANNER + WORKBOOK

	BREAKFAST	LUNCH	DINNER	SNACKS
MONDAY				
TUESDAY				
WEDNESDAY				
THURSDAY				
FRIDAY				
SATURDAY				
SUNDAY				

What will you do if you experience a setback or temptation?
Create a plan for how to get back on track after a dietary slip-up.

....

....

....

....

....

....

Scan the QR code below to get a surprise bonus!

www.ingramcontent.com/pod-product-compliance
Lightning Source LLC
Chambersburg PA
CBHW082108220526
45472CB00009B/2097